YOU'RE NOT CRAZY
IT'S YOUR HORMONES!

THE HORMONE DIVA'S WORKBOOK

YOU'RE NOT CRAZY
IT'S YOUR HORMONES!

THE HORMONE DIVA'S WORKBOOK

Larrian Gillespie

Healthy Life
publications

Visit our website at
http://www.hormonediva.com

Healthy Life Publications Inc.
264 S. La Cienega Blvd., PMB #1233
Beverly Hills, Calif. 90211
1-800-554-3335
1-310-471-2375
1-310-861-5256 FAX

Publisher's Cataloging-in-Publication
(Provided by Quality Books, Inc.)

Gillespie, Larrian.
    You're not crazy it's your hormones!: the hormone
diva's workbook / by Larrian Gillespie
    p. cm.
    Includes bibliographical references and index.
    LCCN 2002114438
    ISBN 0967131766

    1. Endocrine gynecology–Popular works. 2. Hormone
therapy–Popular works. I. Title.

RG159.G55 2003   618.1
                   QB103-200360

Healthy Life Trade Printing: June 2003

Printed in the U.S.A.

10 9 8 7 6 5 4 3 2 1

The information found in this book is from the author's experiences and is not intended to replace medical advice. The author does not directly or indirectly dispense medical advice. This publication is presented for informational purposes only. Before implementing any of the suggestions in this workbook, please consult your physician.

Inside photo: Robert Cavalli, Still Moving Pictures
Book Design by: Barbara Hoorman

Dedication

To Alexian
Always my daughter
now too my friend

and my mother
Dorothy Olive Gillespie

Table of Contents

ACKNOWLEDGMENTS ix

INTRODUCTION:
Be Your Own Health Manager xi

1. Hormone Cycles 1

2. Thyroid Problems 10

3. Adrenal Problems 44

4. Ovarian Problems 62

5. Menopause 96

6. How To Negotiate With Your Doctor 130

7. Charting your Medical Course .146

8. The Hormone Diva Listens 162

9. The Hormone Diva's Survival Kit 182

   Bibliography 198

   Index 206

Acknowledgments

The completion of this workbook would not be possible without the help and encouragement of so many. I dedicate this book:

To Alanna Nash, for being a terrific editor, but more importantly, a great friend.

To Georganne, Ebar and HRH, who never let me get down when things seemed hopeless.

To Emma, one of the most nurturing, loving friends a Diva could have!

To Terri, for being a great web designer and professional advisor.

To my friends, who kept me going despite everything, you are truly important to me.

To Barb Hoorman, for squeezing this project in between dog shows and her "real" work.

To Leslie Blumenberg and Jeanette Leach, PhD, for their help with the thyroid tables.

To all the women on my forums, for challenging the way hormone problems are treated.

Finally, to my family who never believed I was crazy when it was my hormones!

BE YOUR OWN HEALTH MANAGER

If you've ever been frustrated, insulted, patronized or made to feel "hormone" is a dirty word, pull up a chair, because it's time we became good friends.

Let me just start by confirming "you're not crazy" when you can't remember why you walked into a room, or when your hair and skin took on the appearance of someone who's been dragged through a hedge backwards. Hormones exert a powerful effect on every part of our bodies. As a result, when they get out of balance, we exhibit some not-so-subtle responses: sleep disturbance, vaginal dryness, sore gums, joint pain or a swollen stomach.

Unfortunately, in today's HMO time-managed atmosphere, physicians give non life-threatening complaints low priority. If you're female and complain about hormone problems, you're likely to stare into glazed eyeballs followed by "just diet and exercise more" as your doctor scurries out the door. While this advice is certainly important, it doesn't necessarily result in giving you back the glow of a healthy, functioning woman. But you're not doomed to accept the limitations of today's medical system. With a hefty dollop of knowledge, a pinch of guidance and a twist of determination, every woman can learn the secrets to balancing her hormones.

This book is designed to perform as your personal hormone manager, however, it is NOT a complete bible of every hormone problem known to women. The goal is to explain the most common hormonal problems and how to determine which screening studies should be performed to "rule out" a particular diagnosis. I'll begin by explaining the important hormone systems in your body, then show you how to investigate each one to see if it's functioning normally. I'll provide you with a flow chart to document your test results and to record your symptoms as they relate to your menstrual cycle, even in menopause. Need help deciding if certain medications or lab tests are right for your condition? Not to worry. I'll provide you with those answers and the latest scientific articles to support my opinions.

It always helps to know you're not alone in this struggle to achieve better health, so pour yourself a cup of tea and get a shot of sympathy by reading "The Hormone Diva Speaks," a question and answer section culled from my online discussion groups. And if you find that you're still all alone on that healthcare island, I'll give you resources for obtaining diagnostic studies and medications.

Now, more than ever, women need to participate in their healthcare choices if they want to experience a fuller, healthier life. Technology has given the consumer the ability to tap into the same resources available to physicians, expanding their ability to monitor their own health. No longer can women "trust" their doctor has read the vast amount of medical research on hormone therapy and is offering them the best options.

Women instinctively know what is going on with their bodies and deserve advisors who will help serve as interpreters rather than dictators of their health management. "One treatment plan" does not suit all women, especially as they have learned to be cautious about pharmaceutical marketing to both physicians and the public.

It's time to take control.

HORMONE CYCLES

1

HORMONE CYCLES

Every woman is a hormone diva, a goddess, endowed with the ability to create life through the power of hormones. Unfortunately, when those little suckers fly out of control, we can morph into head-spinning demons. So, in order to figure out which ones would benefit from a little gentle coaxing back in line, you need to understand the hormone game.

THE RULES

Hormones must play well with others. They must be able to share, not hog, receptors on cell membranes, and sometimes they need a little "time out" in order to keep their excitement level in control during your menstrual cycle. A tiny gland behind your eyes, the hypothalamus, acts as the umpire directing all the action. She rides on the back of the pituitary, your pitcher.

THE NORMAL CYCLE

Let's follow what happens during a normal menstrual cycle. Day 1 is the first day you bleed. As you can see, your body temperature is around 36.2 degrees centigrade, or about 98.6. (see Figure 1) Your progesterone level (P) has bottomed out because pregnancy did not occur. Estradiol (E2), the active form

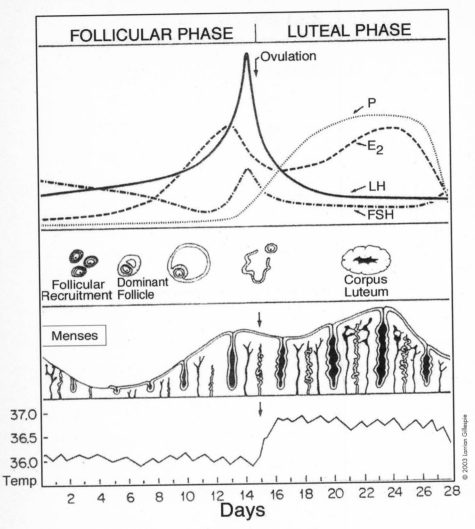

Figure 1 **The normal menstrual cycle**

of estrogen, is also low at this time. The uterine lining is beginning to shed, but really doesn't reach its lowest level until days 5-7. This is known as the pre-follicular stage, as the ovary

Menstrual Cycle

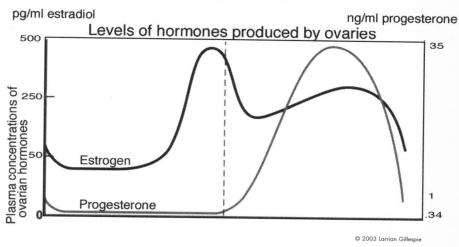

pg/ml estradiol

ng/ml progesterone

Levels of hormones produced by ovaries

Figure 2 **Hormonal levels throughout a normal cycle**

© 2003 Larrian Gillespie

has yet to choose the next egg up to bat. Around Day 10 the selected egg goes into training. Estradiol levels start to rise and a big cheer goes up when leutenizing hormone (LH), along with follicle stimulating hormone (FSH), spike the egg into ovulation. This ends the follicular phase. The luteal phase begins with a rise in your body temp in response to Progesterone (P), the designated hitter, taking over and running the bases, along with estradiol, for a double play. The uterine lining builds up, ready for implantation. If fertilization has not occurred, both hormones get tagged out and the uterine lining begins to shed.

Throughout this book you will find the following symbols:

**Scroll symbol
represents laboratory results**

**This symbol means
"see your doctor"**

**This symbol
represents medication**

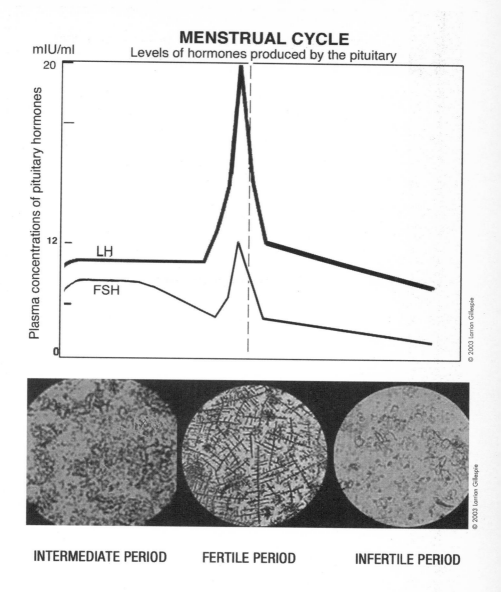

Figure 3 **Ferning pattern seen with ovulation using a sialic acid tester**

THE ABNORMAL CYCLE

So what happens when your cycle isn't a classic 28 days? The answer lies in the follicular phase. In perimenopause, the LH surge moves up a few days, shortening your cycle by 2-3 days. If the LH surge is delayed or there is not sufficient estradiol and FSH to spike ovulation, your cycle may lengthen to 32 days or even longer. The luteal phase remains constant at 14 days regardless of the behavior of the follicular phase.[1]

Now take a look at the hormones produced by the ovaries. (see Figure 2) Notice that estrogen should be no lower than 200 pg/ml between days 13 and 15. Progesterone should always be low in the first half of your cycle, because it's the ovulated egg that stimulates progesterone production. If you don't ovulate, your progesterone levels will be low in the second half, as will your basal temperature reading.

How do you know if you've ovulated? Here's a great little secret "old time" docs used to determine ovulation before blood tests were available.

During ovulation (Days 11-14) estrogen increases the amount of potassium chloride and sialic acid (neuraminic acid) in your saliva. Crystals form a unique "fern" pattern when your saliva is dried on glass, making it simple to determine if you have actually ovulated.[2-4] (see Figure 3) This test is 90% accurate even in non-medical hands. In Chapter Nine I will tell you how to obtain a sialic acid tester as part of your Hormone Diva Survival Kit.

Charting your symptoms as they relate to your menstrual cycle is important. Hormone divas simply have too much on their minds to trust their memories. So I've made a simple chart that will keep your important observations accurate. I've placed a master copy of this chart in Chapter 7 so you'll always have a new one for each month. Since no two hormone divas have the identical complaints, I've left space for you to put in any symptoms unique to your cycle. Remember Day 1 is the first day you bleed. Rank your symptoms each day using 1 for no symptoms, 2 for mild, 3 for moderately severe and 4 for "feels like hell." You'll see the pattern in no time this way.

		SIALIC ACID POS	FOOD CRAVINGS	INSOMNIA	HEADACHE	FATIGUE	BACKACHE	ACHES/PAINS	CRAMPING	ABD BLOATING	BREAST TENDER	SWOLLEN FEET	SWOLLEN HANDS	CRYING SPELL	ANGER	ANXIETY	DEPRESSION	DAY OF CYCLE
																		1
																		2
																		3
																		4
																		5
																		6
																		7
																		8
																		9
																		10
																		11
																		12
																		13
																		14
																		15
																		16
																		17
																		18
																		19
																		20
																		21
																		22
																		23
																		24
																		25
																		26
																		27
																		28
																		29
																		30
																		31

Rank your symptoms each day. 1=no symptoms   2=mild   3=moderately severe   4="feels like hell"

Table 1 **Chart for menstrual symptoms**

Now that you have a firm grasp of "what's normal," I'm going to show you how the other team players can throw a hormonal foul ball your way. Their lineup is composed of thyroid, adrenal, and ovarian disorders than can knock your fast pitch out of the ballpark. In order to help you figure out their strategy, I'm going to start with a relevant quiz in each section, so sharpen your pencils.

2

THYROID PROBLEMS

Let's start by looking at your menstrual cycle chart. Do you have more than five symptoms marked with a score of 3 or higher for several days at a time? If so, your hormones definitely need some adjusting.

Funky hormones may spark the occasional urge to **P**ummel **M**en's **S**crotums, but unrecognized thyroid problems can turn any fun loving diva into a pugilist. So here's your first quiz to help decide if your thyroid is a prime suspect in your hormonal behavior. Now, before you take this test, I really think you need to view it somewhat like reading your horoscope. It can be entertaining, even educating, but don't plan your life by it. The same information can apply to other organs, **so the findings are not conclusive you MUST have a thyroid problem.** I intentionally did not list every symptom known to woman. Anyone who has been diagnosed with thyroid problems in the past already knows her gland has a record of misbehavior. So, ready to grill your suspect hormone? Let's turn up the heat with a few probing questions.

A Word About Test Ranges

Lab reports were designed to be so easy to read any elevator operator could understand them, but it takes basic medical knowledge to interpret the significance of values within those ranges. Unfortunately, office personnel and even some doctors hold to the theory that a lab value is "normal" if they don't put a little warning flag by it. No wonder women hear "everything's fine" as the doctor quickly runs his or her finger down the page and scoots out the door.

As numerous companies manufacture testing assays, the ranges for a normal lab value may be completely different depending upon which laboratory kit is purchased. To make matters worse, each hormone may have a different unit value, such as pmol/L or iU/ml. Furthermore, outdated standards are used by laboratories, bracketing a TSH between .45 and 5 as "normal." However, a recent study of the US population narrows that range considerably. TSH values between 1-1.5 and a total T4 near 112 should now be considered "normal."[5]

YOU MIGHT HAVE A THYROID PROBLEM IF

- You gain weight "magically" despite diet and exercise
- You are constipated most of the time
- You feel tired, run down, exhausted
- You feel cold when others are hot
- Your hair is brittle, coarse and falling out
- Your nails crack, break easily
- You're losing the hair from the outer margins of your eyebrows
- You have longer, heavier, crampier or more frequent periods
- Your skin is dry, scaly and looks like the Mojave Desert
- You feel depressed
- You have trouble sleeping and snore like a lawnmower
- Your sex drive makes you a candidate for virgin recertification
- You feel something is stuck in your throat
- Your memory is changing...what memory?
- Your eyes are sensitive to light

If you answered yes to eight or more of these questions, you need to pursue your investigation of thyroid misconduct. However, first you need to understand how your thyroid gland functions.

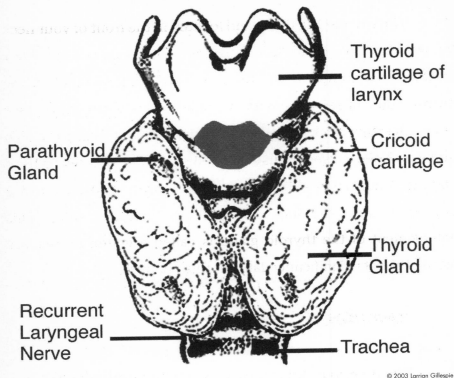

Thyroid cartilage of larynx

Cricoid cartilage

Parathyroid Gland

Thyroid Gland

Recurrent Laryngeal Nerve

Trachea

© 2003 Larrian Gillespie

Figure 4 **Anatomy of the thyroid gland**

LOCATION

The thyroid is a tiny gland located in the front of your neck below your "Adam's apple". It has two lobes that straddle your trachea or windpipe. If you tip your head back and look in the mirror, you can see their butterfly shape quite easily. Now place your fingertips over each lobe and feel for any bumps, called nodules. None present? That's a good sign. Now bring your head back to a normal position. Look again at your thyroid. Does it appear you're sporting a sausage on either side? This enlargement of the thyroid gland is called a goiter. I'll tell you more about its significance later in this chapter.

FUNCTION

The thyroid gland is the diva of metabolism, which proves powerful things come in small packages. Like a slave, your thyroid works endlessly to combine teeny tiny amounts of iodine with an amino acid, called tyrosine, in order to make triiodothyronine (T3) and thyroxine (T4). These hormones are responsible for converting calories and oxygen into energy for every cell in your body. T4 makes up about 90% of your thyroid gland's production, but T3 possesses about five times the hormone strength of T4. Your liver and kidneys convert T4 into T3 and its inert component, reverse T3.

Remember the pituitary, our hormonal star pitcher? When the level of T3 and T4 drops too low, the hypothalamus suggests via TSH Releasing Hormone (TRH), the pituitary call for a special play. This involves Thyroid Stimulating Hormone (TSH), which gives your thyroid gland a much-needed charge as it runs the bases. Up goes the production of T3 and T4 until normal levels are reached. Your team has scored!

STEEERIKE!

Like any game, there are several ways to strike out. The pitcher might misread the signals and wave off TSH or the bases could be loaded, preventing the conversion of T4 into T3. Antibodies could attack the thyroid with a foul ball. So in order to obtain all the correct information, you need to test for central regulation (pituitary/hypothalamic axis, i.e. TSH), peripheral conversion (T4 to T3) and autoimmune involvement (antibodies).

LAB PATTERNS IN THYROID ILLNESS

	TSH	FT4	FT3	rT3	α-TPO	α-Tg
Early Hashimoto	nl	nl	nl	nl	±	⇧
Late Hashimoto	⇧	⇩	⇩	±	⇧	±
Early Graves	⇩	nl	⇧	±	⇧	⇧
Late Graves	⇩	⇧	⇧	⇧	⇧	±
Low T3, or ESS (Wilson's syndrome)	nl	nl	⇩	⇧	-	-

© 2003 Larrian Gillespie

TSH=thyroid stimulating hormone FT4=free FT3=free rT3=reverse α=antibodies
TPO=thyroid peroxidase TG=thyroglobulin ESS=Euthyroid Sick Syndrome

Table 2 **Lab values for thyroid conditions**

HASHIMOTO'S THYROIDITIS

In 1912 Japanese researcher Dr. Hakaru Hashimoto discovered white blood cells were sneaking into the thyroid gland, causing inflammation, swelling and eventually scarring the

Monica's story

Monica was only 37 but felt as if she was over the hill. She was tired, irritable and unable to give her husband and little girl the attention they deserved. Her hair, which had once been long and glossy, was falling out in clumps. Even her eyebrows had taken on a peculiar alien look all their own. "I could have passed as Mr. Spock's sister , since I only had half an eyebrow anymore. I noticed my face seemed puffy but I really thought something was wrong when I could barely lift my daughter, who only weighed twenty pounds. I felt weak. When my family was out of the house, I would turn the heat up, because my hands and feet were always cold. I even went to bed with socks on my feet. Worst of all, I couldn't sleep. My periods, which had been regular as clockwork, became heavy and lasted longer than before. When I told my doctor all this, she said I was "depressed" and gave me a sample of some antidepressant medication. It didn't help and it really made me gain weight. I knew something was wrong, but I wasn't getting any help. My husband started searching on the internet, and all my symptoms made us suspicious I was hypothyroid. I went back to my doctor, but she said my blood tests were "normal" and dismissed me. So did the next three doctors I visited. Finally, I decided to take matters into my own hands and demanded a referral to an endocrinologist who specialized in thyroid problems. He agreed to try me on medication even though my labs were "normal." I began to feel like my old self again. It took some adjusting of doses, but now I look AND feel my age again."

tissue. This condition is the most common reason for low thyroid function or hypothyroidism, especially in women. As a result, the body brings in its defense team, called antibodies, to seal up the leaks with nature's "super glue" — fibrinogen. The presence of antibodies to thyroid peroxidase (TPO), an enzyme, develops whenever there is cellular leakage from your thyroid. Thyroglobulin (TG) is a large protein manufactured in response to TSH stimulation. T4 is produced when tyrosine molecules in TG are combined with iodine as a result of TPO.

Symptoms of hypothyroidism include constipation, depression, weight gain, heavy bleeding during a period, sleeping problems such as sleep apnea, hair loss, dry skin and nails and a low sex drive, just to name a few. Your thyroid gland may become swollen but not especially tender. Women are frequently underdiagnosed for reasons that would pull the hair out of any diva's head: failure to recognize thyroid problems as the leading cause for gynecologic complaints.

Trust me on this one. It's not a conspiracy, but rather the result of subspecialization in medicine. "Female problems" have been compartmentalized under the domain of gynecology and only recently has the sub-subspecialty of reproductive endocrinology appeared. But if you don't want a test tube baby, all other fertility related problems are left in the hands of the "general" gynecologist who only knows about "birthing them babies." So it's up to you to raise the issue of possible thyroid problems.

GRAVES' DISEASE

Is your heart thumping like a xylophone in your chest? Graves' disease, or hyperthyroidism, is an autoimmune problem that occurs seven times more frequently in women than men. Like Hashimoto's thyroiditis, a goiter may develop, but it's tender, even painful to your touch. Although you might develop "bug eyes" (exophthalmos) from too much thyroid hormone, symptoms of muscle weakness, anxiety or nervousness (can we say panic attacks?) and exhaustion are far more common. Your marauding immune system may even paint a bull's eye on your ovaries, causing changes in your menstrual cycle, resulting in premature menopause. One thing is clear: hyperthyroidism can kill you if left undiagnosed. So, let's take another quiz.

YOU MIGHT BE HYPERTHYROID IF

- Your pulse rate could pass for a jackhammer on speed
- Your appetite rivals The Rock but you're losing weight
- You avoid hot drinks because your hands shake too much
- Sweat pours off you like a racehorse at the finish line
- Your reflexes have the tone of a taut rubber band
- You've taken up designer sheep counting instead of sleep
- You feel weak as a kitten but roar like a lion at little things
- Your bowels have more movements than a Beethoven concerto
- You constantly hear ringing in your ears
- Your periods are as scarce as Sharon Stone's underpants
- Your hair is dry, brittle and falling out
- You feel like elephants are sitting on your chest
- You feel dizzy, faint or about to fall down
- You've become a collector of wrinkle creams
- Your toes keep crossing and cramping
- Your moods change faster than a DSL screen

Unlike hypothyroidism, hyperthyroid conditions wreak havoc by elevating your blood pressure and interfering with the electrical conduction or rhythm of your heart. This can lead to heart failure and even sudden death.

Delores's Story

The year 2001 was stressful for Delores. "I lost my job to downsizing and it was difficult finding a new position. I had always been a confident person, but now I was trembling, feeling short of breath, and unable to sleep. I just picked at my food. I lost ten pounds without any effort, but I didn't feel well. I knew something was wrong. I have a great family doctor, but even he thought my symptoms must be a combination of stress and menopause. One night, I experienced my first panic attack and ended up in the emergency room. The doctor was amazed at my pulse rate, which was over 120 beats. He felt my neck and decided to run thyroid studies. He told me I was hyperthyroid, but I didn't believe him, because I didn't have bulging eyes. He explained that I had a swollen thyroid gland, called a goiter, which stood out even more since my weight loss. That night was the beginning of my new life. I'm on a combination of medications, and feel that I'm going to get well."

Think hyperthyroidism is easy to recognize? Just ask Olympic Gold Medallist Gail Devers, who was undiagnosed for two years despite severe weight loss, heart problems, dry skin, fatigue, and impending baldness. Doctors were so clueless as to the cause of her symptoms they even recommended amputation of her feet! And don't let them dismiss your complaints because you don't have "bug eyes" or have gained weight. Protruding eyeballs occur in only a small percentage of patients. Hyperthyroidism can cause insulin resistance, which results in weight gain, not weight loss. If you suspect you might be hyperthyroid, concentrate on getting the right tests done.

EUTHYROID SICK SYNDROME

Stress, especially sudden severe stress, may cause your body to release "fight or flight" chemicals that can block the ability of your tissues to convert T4 into T3. Gangs of inflammatory chemicals, called cytokines, appear to be the troublemakers, knocking out your pituitary and hypothalamus' intricate regulatory mechanisms. One subtle indication of "foul play" is your body temperature. The hypothalamus is responsible for raising it in the afternoon and keeping it low during the evening and morning hours. Now imagine nasty cytokines throwing dust into the umpire's eyes, making her unable to signal your body temperature to "do the wave." As a result, everyone stays in her seat and your temperature fails to display a nice up and down pattern.

Don't shoot your thyroid for being the messenger in this kind of situation! Finding a low Free T3, normal T4, and "normal" TSH plus low body temperature readings indicates the problem is coming from elsewhere in your body.[6] Start checking out your adrenal glands, ovaries, hypothalamus, pituitary, kidneys, liver, or bowel. Once you find and treat the cause, your thyroid will return to being a happy camper again.

TREATMENT OPTIONS

Hypothyroidism is perhaps one of the most misunderstood conditions in the medical lexicon of diseases, largely due to the drug literature from pharmaceutical companies. The manufacturers of T4 supplements have told doctors they only need to replace T4 in order to restore "normal" thyroid function. This would be fine if the only cause for hypothyroidism was a failure to produce enough T4. Of course, all the research studies were done in men, who have very low estradiol levels, no fluctuating hormone cycles, different liver enzymes, a lower incidence of adrenal problems and oodles of tyrosine available in comparison to women. It's a no-brainer that women recognized simply swallowing a pill didn't spin hormonal straw into gold. When research was recently done in females, the results were quite different from advertised.

Many women, but not all, need both T3 and T4 supplementation if they want to feel like a goddess again. T3 was found to greatly improve a woman's mood, especially if she suffers from depression or irritability. It can even sharpen our capacity to recognize objects and remember where the keys are hiding.[7]

And don't forget about your stomach. Just because you swallow a tablet doesn't mean you're breaking it down completely. Hormone changes affect your entire metabolic processing plant. Progesterone slows down gastric emptying by holding food and medication an hour longer in the upper or first part of your stomach.[8] Too much or too little gastric acid can interfere with the breakdown of the talc used to make a tablet. Hormone imbalances may even affect the enzymes in your liver, resulting in lower blood values than expected from a dose of medication. And don't leave out your blood sugar levels. Swings in glucose from Type 2 Diabetes can make regulating your medication a nightmare.

GENERIC	BRANDS	CONTAINS	RATIO
Levothyroxine (synthetic)	Synthroid Eltroxin Levoxyl Levothyroid Unithroid	T4, thyroxine	100%
Liothyronine (synthetic)	Cytomel	T3, triidodothyronine	100%
Liotrix (synthetic)	Thyrolar	T4/T3	50%T4 50%T3* bioactive
Natural thyroid (derived from pig thyroid)	Armour Thyroid Westhroid Naturethroid	T4/T3/T2/T1 Nonspecific Animal factors	51%T4 48%T3* bioactive

*T3 is 4 times as potent as T4 on a microgram to microgram basis

Table 3 **Thyroid medications**

By now you're starting to understand why a hormone diva has to monitor her medication's effectiveness with blood tests. Just because you swallow a pill doesn't mean your body is getting the most out of it. Even the type of thyroid hormone you receive from your doctor needs to be scrutinized, as frankly, many doctors prescribe "out of habit" the brand they are most familiar with in their practice.

Now, remember the body "naturally" produces a ratio of 90% T4 to 10% T3 by weight. As you can see, none of the above medications "mimic" this ratio, offering too much or no T3 at all. (see Table 3) No wonder women can have a normal TSH value on medication, but feel like they're wandering around in a fog. So how do you add T3 to your treatment plan?

MEDICATION ALGEBRA

Translating your current T4 prescription into a combination T3/T4 combo might require a mathematical wizard to figure it out correctly. However, I've pulled together some tables to get you rolling. You'll notice that obtaining precisely 10% T3 is tougher than you think, because we're limited by the pill sizes manufactured today. So, let's start by aiming as close as possible without the need for magnifying loops, weight scales and surgical instruments.

Your doctor will probably start you on T4 medication. We can calculate the equivalence of 1 mcg T3= 4 mcg T4. If you want to add T3 (using Cytomel), just check out Table 4.

A WORD ABOUT THE THUMPIES

If you feel an overwhelming sense of fear while your heart plays "Baba Lou" in your chest, you may be experiencing a panic attack. Erratic production of thyroid hormone can create "storms", which will throw around your emotions, blood pressure and heart rate better than a typhoon. Too much thyroid medication can produce the same results, making you feel anxious, short of breath, and preoccupied with an overwhelming sense of doom. As you might expect, changes in thyroid hormone production can also lower your estradiol levels once your adrenals start pumping out cortisol and adrenaline. And if you suffer from a mild mitral valve condition, called insufficiency or prolapse, you just won the pink elephant at the panic attack carnival. So what can you do?

• Make sure your TSH is above .5 and your T3 is not riding the rocket to the upper level.

• Try some estradiol to help counter the elevated thyroid hormone production. Estrace .5mg or 1/2 stick of estrogel should be adequate.

• Mix 1/2 teaspoon of baking soda in water and drink it JUST ONCE. When you experience a panic attack, your body becomes acidotic from your rapid breathing and baking soda will help to rebalance your system.

• Tagamet 200mg can also slow down a nerve signaling pathway behind the duodenum that sends messages to your heart to race like a thoroughbred at the Kentucky Derby.

• Inderal, a beta blocker, can also prevent your heart from winning the rhumba contest.

Current Dose	Equivalent T4 plus T3 (Exact)		Closest approximation by full tablets			
T4 dose (mcg)	T4 (mcg)	T3 (mcg)	Synthetic T4	Synthetic T3	T4 equivalent	Actual % T3
50	34.6	3.8	25	5	45	17%
75	51.9	5.8	50	5	70	9%
87	60.2	6.7	75	5	95	6%
100	69.2	7.7	75	10	105	12%
112	77.5	8.6	75	10	115	12%
125	86.5	9.6	87	10	127	10%
150	103.8	11.5	100	10	140	9%
200	138.5	15.4	137	15	197	10%
300	207.7	23.1	200	25	300	11%

Table 4

If you want to verify these figures, divide your T4 dose by 13. This will give you the amount of T3 for proper balance. Multiply the value by 9 for the T4 level.

THYROID ANTIBODIES AND SELENIUM

In a recent study, researchers discovered that a deficiency of selenium can reduce the activity of glutathione peroxidase, an enzyme that has numerous effects on the immune system. It can also alter the conversion of T4 to T3, as the deiodinase enzyme is selenium dependent. Patients who received 200mcg of sodium selenite daily reduced their thyroid antibodies by 60%.[11]

Natural sources of selenium include:
- Brazil nuts
- tuna
- oysters
- turkey
- chicken
- wheat germ
- brown rice
- oatmeal
- eggs

Thyrolar: Achieving 10% T3 with Thyrolar is possible, but again, you are limited by the finite sizes of Thyrolar available.(see Table 5)

Current T4 dose	Thyrolar	T4	T3%
50 mcg	.25	25 mcg	10%
100 mcg	.50	50 mcg	10%
200 mcg	1	100 mcg	10%
300 mcg	1.5	150 mcg	10%

Table 5

Armour thyroid: 1 grain (60 mg) of Armour thyroid contains 38 mcg of T4 and 9 mcg of T3. (19% T3 and 81% T4). If you calculate using the formula of 1 mcg T3 = 4 mcg T4, then 1 grain is equivalent to 74 mcg of T4. However, the manufacturer (Forrest Pharmaceutical) provides equivalence information showing that 1 grain of Armour is equivalent to 100 mcg of T4. So, Table 6 for achieving 10% T3 is calculated using the amount of T3 in Armour, but assuming the total is 100 mcg T4 equivalent.

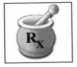

Current T4 dose	Armour (grains)	T4 (mcg)	% T3
25	1/8	12.5	8%
50	1/4	25	8%
100	1/2	50	8%
125	3/4	50	12%
150	3/4	75	8%
200	1	100	8%
300	1 1/2	150	8%

Table 6

Now I see glazed eyeballs here. Just realize, these calculations are a starting point for getting near a 10% T3 level. Be aware, everyone is unique in their metabolic profile, so you may require some tweaking of your medication to feel your best.

There are numerous combinations possible, such as adding pure T3 to pure T4. However, T3 needs to be in a sustained or slow release formula in order to prevent a severe case of the "thumpies" from occurring. So, how do you know if your medication is making a change in the right direction?

RETESTING YOUR LEVELS

If you've started medication, or just changed the brand, it only takes about 21 days for blood levels to stabilize. You should have repeat testing of the entire thyroid panel until your values are within range. After that, twice a year testing is recommended, as your thyroid medication needs differ seasonally. You may need more thyroid medication in the winter or cold months, and less in the summer or warmer months of the year.[9] And don't forget to retest your levels if you begin hormone replacement therapy or birth control pills. Estrogen can affect a protein that binds

SYMPTOMS OF LOW FERRITIN

- Depression
- Fatigue
- Listlessness
- Impaired learning
- Poor memory
- Decreased attention span
- Irritability
- Dizziness
- Appetite loss
- Constipation
- Difficulty swallowing
- Joint soreness
- Asthma
- Sores on skin
- Hair loss
- Headaches
- Sore or burning tongue
- Brittle, flat, or spoon shaped nails
- Longitudinal ridges on nails
- Heart palpitations on exertion
- Shortness of breath
- Cold extremities
- Decreased resistance to infection
- Anemia (hypochromic, microcytic)
- Numbness & tingling
- Night sweats
- Fragile bones
- Growth impairment
- Eye soreness

DO NOT SUPPLEMENT WITH IRON UNLESS YOU HAVE A SERUM FERRITIN TEST THAT SHOWS A VALUE LESS THAN 100. Do not take more than 20mg of elemental iron a day as it depletes zinc.

thyroxine, lowering your blood values by almost 20%.[10]

Problems getting your levels under control? You could be anemic. Iron stores in the body are reflected as serum ferritin, which affects the production of red blood cells in the body. It also affects your blood insulin levels. Iron deficiency anemia lowers thyroid peroxidase (TPO) activity, a heme-containing enzyme important in thyroid hormone synthesis.[12] If you are hypothyroid and anemic, you won't be able to adjust your levels properly until the anemia is corrected, usually with liquid ferrous sulfate. If you are hyperthyroid, you might have too much serum ferritin in your body, which can interfere with your medication. Simply donating blood once a month can be enough to bring your insulin, ferritin and thyroid levels under control.[13] Undiagnosed adrenal insufficiency can also cause problems with your thyroid medication.[14] In the next chapter, I will show you how to discover if you have this condition.

Like iron, swings in your blood sugar can also make stabilizing your medication difficult. With the epidemic of Type 2 diabetes caused by obesity, it is important your doctor know your blood sugar and insulin levels if you want to keep your TSH levels in control.[15]

FOOD NOT TO BE EATEN RAW
— MAY BE USED COOKED

- cabbage
- kale
- kohlrabi
- rutabaga
- cauliflower
- mustard greens
- radishes
- broccoli
- brussel sprouts
- corn
- peas
- lima beans
- sweet potatoes
- cassava
- sorghum
- apricots
- prunes
- walnuts
- cherries
- almonds
- soybeans
- bamboo shoots

BORDERLINE HYPOTHYROIDISM THERAPY

As we divas "mature", the tendency to develop hypothyroidism increases each year, especially after our ovaries go two claws up. However, there are several dietary ways to manage a borderline thyroid without medication by avoiding the following:

• **Soy:** Isoflavones, found in soy products and supplements, interfere with thyroid and estrogen receptors, lowering your levels of these hormones. Just 30 mg of isoflavones can send your thyroid into shutdown by blocking thyroid peroxidase enzymes and stimulating anti-thyroid antibodies.[16] They can disrupt your menstrual cycle, cause infertility and wreck havoc with your hormones for several months.[17] Isoflavones, especially those in supplements, can even lower your sex drive.[18]

• **Iodinated Salt:** Iodine, found in seaweed wraps and table salt, can lower your thyroid function, causing your tissue to swell up like a puffer fish at a whistling contest.[19,20,21] Avoid sushi with kelp wraps and use natural sea salt, which contains numerous minerals and just a trace of iodine.

- **Goitrogenic Vegetables:** Raw vegetables, such as broccoli, cabbage, rutabaga, parsnips, radishes, cauliflower, kale and soybeans, can act like antithyroid drugs, tipping the function of your borderline thyroid gland into low gear.[22, 23]

- **High Glycemic Carbohydrates:** Consuming carbohydrates such as sugar, corn, bleached flour products, pastas, breads, rice and cereals, raises insulin levels and cortisol in your body. This adrenal hormone acts to suppress TSH and can block conversion of T4 to T3.[24]

- **Lack of Exercise:** Failure to exercise on a routine basis affects the peripheral conversion of T4 to T3, as seen in the Euthyroid Sick Syndrome and Chronic Fatigue Syndrome.[25, 26] Although I believe that, if God had wanted divas to exercise She would have strewn the floor with diamonds, any consistent choice of exercise will help keep your thyroid gland sparkling around your neck.

TREATMENT OF HYPERTHYROIDISM

As you might guess, this condition requires expert management with medication, radioactive iodine (RAI), or surgery. However, recent links between RAI use and subsequent breast cancer has made this approach much less desirable.[27] Anti-thyroid medications, such as propylthiouracil (PTU) or methimazole (Tapazole) block your thyroid gland's ability to use iodine, which lowers your thyroid hormone levels. Finally, surgery to remove the thyroid gland results in converting a hyperthyroid patient gradually into a hypothyroid one, so it's important to check your TSH levels every six months after surgery. Remember, hyperthyroidism can kill you, so demand to be under the care of a thyroid specialist and not a general practitioner.

THYROID NODULES

Feeling a lump in your thyroid gland would give anyone concern. However, let me give you a few guidelines regarding thyroid nodules. They are perhaps the most common kind of "lump" detectable by your hands. One in twelve to fifteen women have thyroid nodules. Almost all of them are non-cancerous, because most are the result of encapsulation of normal thyroid tissue, or filled with fluid, such as a cyst. These little buggers, however, can be very hormonally active.

The first step, once a nodule has been detected, is to have thyroid lab studies done and an ultrasound. The ultrasound will

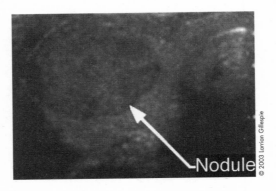

© 2003 Larrian Gillespie

Figure 5 **Thyroid nodule seen on ultrasound**

allow your doctor to determine if the nodule is working like the Lone Ranger or has a posse of other nodules.

The next step is a thyroid scan. Since thyroid tissue needs iodine to make thyroxine, a radioactive isotope containing iodine is injected into your vein to determine if the nodule is actively making thyroid hormone. A "hot" nodule is one that is making MORE thyroxine than the rest of your thyroid gland and will show up darker than the surrounding tissue. This is seen frequently with hyperthyroidism. A "cold" nodule appears as a light area when compared to the rest of your thyroid tissue, and may represent a cyst or benign adenoma. Only fifteen percent of cold nodules are cancerous.[28]

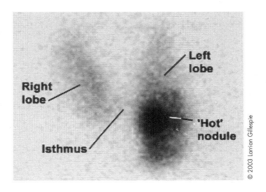

Figure 6 **Hot nodule seen on thyroid isotope scan**

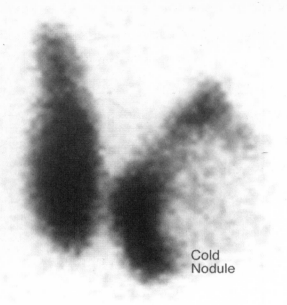

Cold
Nodule

© 2003 Lorrian Gillespie

Figure 7 **Cold nodule on thyroid scan.
Notice how it appears white due to lack of uptake
of the radioactive iodine.**

The only way to determine if it represents a malignancy is to have a fine needle aspiration biopsy done. This extracts cells so the pathologist can check them for malignancy.

Now that you have an understanding of your thyroid gland, let's move on to an important pair of glands that sit right above your kidneys: The adrenal glands.

ADRENAL PROBLEMS

3

Stress, both physical and emotional, can only be tolerated if your adrenal glands are holding down the fortress. Shaped like pyramids, these powerhouses sit on top of your kidneys, which are located under your rib cage, high up near your bra line. (Surprised at their location? No wonder a "kidney belt," which is worn around the lower back by boxers, offers little protection!)

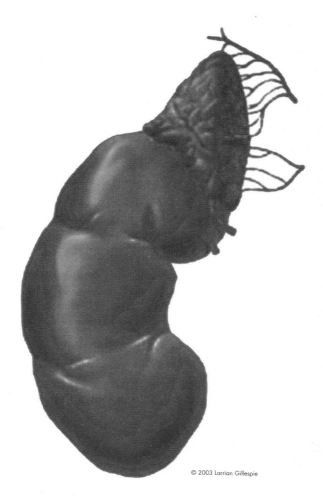

© 2003 Larrian Gillespie

Figure 8 **Kidney with the adrenal gland riding on top**

Each gland is composed of two parts: The outer region is called the adrenal cortex and the inner area the medulla. Your adrenal glands must work synchronously with your pituitary and hypothalamus to release steroids and other hormones that regulate your blood pressure and salt balance.

The cortex produces the following hormones *(see Figure 9):*

• Corticosteroids

> • hydrocortisone (cortisol) which tells your body how to use fats, proteins and carbohydrates.

> • corticosterone, which works with cortisol to shut down inflammatory reactions in the body which affect your immune system. Cortisol is produced in a rhythmic diurnal or 12 hour cycle, with the highest levels released around 3 — 4 AM and a small amount again around 4PM. The adrenals produce essentially no cortisol between 6PM — 3AM.

> • aldosterone, which together with renin and angiotensin, helps to regulate your blood pressure by regulating the amount of sodium lost in urine.

- androgenic steroids, such as testosterone, DHEA, pregnenolone and progesterone.

The medulla is the guardian of one's ability to cope with stress. It secretes

- Epinephrine (adrenaline), which increases your heart rate, directs blood preferentially to the brain and heart, and tells the liver to manufacture glucose for extra energy needs.

- norepinephrine (noradrenaline), which stimulates peripheral constriction of blood vessels, such as those in your fingertips, skin and stomach, in order to increase your blood pressure so you don't faint under stress.

The release of these neurotransmitters from the medulla is under the control of the autonomic nervous system. Sympathetic nerves located in the medulla can dump significant amounts of epinephrine into the blood stream when we are frightened or experience a panic attack. They can also make fine adjustments in our blood pressure by releasing norepinephrine when we go from lying down to an upright position. These same nerves fine tune our reaction to stresses in our environment, such as excessive vibration, changes in altitude and barometric pressure, temperature or humidity. So, how do you know if your adrenal glands are working as they should?

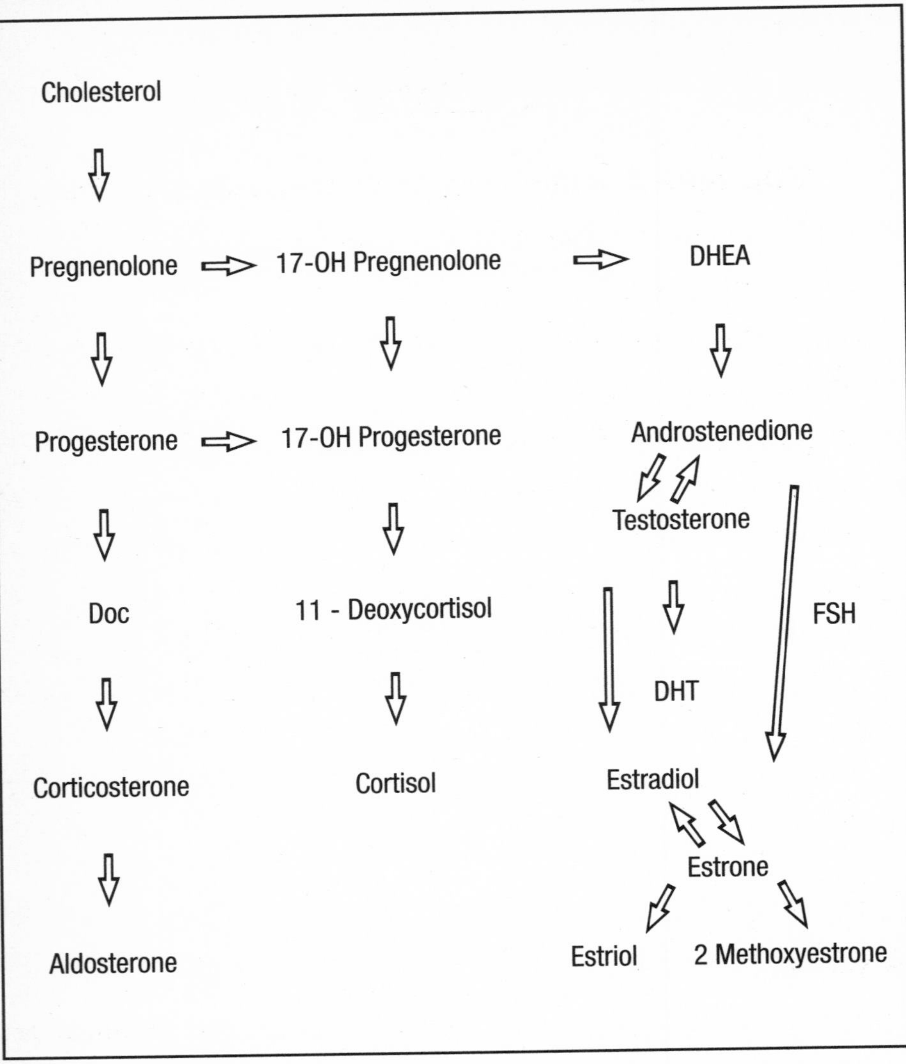

Cholesterol

⇩

Pregnenolone ⇒ 17-OH Pregnenolone ⇒ DHEA

⇩ ⇩ ⇩

Progesterone ⇒ 17-OH Progesterone Androstenedione

⇩ ⇩ ⇗⇗
Testosterone

Doc 11 - Deoxycortisol FSH

⇩ ⇩ ⇩

Corticosterone Cortisol DHT

⇩ Estradiol

Aldosterone ⇗⇘
Estrone

⇗ ⇘
Estriol 2 Methoxyestrone

Figure 9 **Synthesis of adrenal hormones**

YOU MIGHT HAVE LOW ADRENAL FUNCTION IF (ADDISON'S DISEASE)

• Scars take on a brown stain and your joints, lips and skin folds or creases, such as on the palms of your hands, appear "dirty"

• You challenge the deer for the salt lick

• You run a strange low grade fever, especially around four in the afternoon

• You feel tired all the time

• You just can't seem to shake that "flu-like" feeling

• You can fall asleep at the drop of a hat, but you never feel rested

• You can't "jump out of bed" without becoming dizzy or faint

• Depression and "brain fog" have become your constant companion

• The room is always too hot or too cold

• The slightest noise has you jumping out of your skin

• Your pubic hair is so thin it needs a "comb-over"

• You become hypoglycemic and start to shake within a few hours after eating

• You crave black licorice or licorice root to keep from feeling "light headed"

Orthostatic hypotension

One of the most sensitive tests for primary adrenal insufficiency is to measure systolic blood pressure lying down, then suddenly sitting upright. If the reclining blood pressure is <110 and drops, rather than rises when sitting up, one should suspect adrenal insufficiency. Aldosterone and renin levels should be measured supine (lying down) and erect (sitting up) in this instance, as a single level will be the "average" of this response and appear normal. Low serum sodium levels and elevated potassium values complete the picture.

If you answered yes to more than five of these symptoms, you may have damage to your adrenal glands called Addison's disease. Now this condition has several levels, or degrees of damage. Primary adrenal insufficiency (true Addison's Disease) is due to direct damage to the adrenal tissue. It presents with both an inability to regulate your sodium and potassium levels and very low cortisol/sex hormone levels. The original cause was a fungus, such as tuberculosis. The major cause of adrenal insufficiency in our society is a defect in the immune system. Stress, especially chronic stress, can overexcite the sympathetic nerve pathways in the medulla, decreasing blood supply to the tissue. This causes a breakdown in the protective barrier of the cell, exposing the intracellular elements to toxins and free radicals circulating in the lymph and blood. Almost 90% of the adrenal gland has to be damaged before the clinical symptoms of Addison's disease are easily recognized.[29]

Secondary adrenal insufficiency (AI) is caused by a defect in the signaling mechanism from the pituitary. This results in low levels of ACTH (adrenocorticotrophic hormone), which signals the release of cortisol from the adrenals. As you might guess, viruses and pituitary lesions (hemorrhages) or tumors can cause this problem. Tertiary (3rd degree) AI results from inadequate cortisol releasing hormone (CRH) responses. The usual presentation of both these defects is low levels of the androgenic or male hormones and cortisol. Because ACTH is decreased, there is no "tell tale" brown staining of the skin. Salt balance remains normal as well.

The sneaky thing about adrenal insufficiency, regardless of its cause, is the gradual nature of the beast. It starts out with partial hormonal changes in cortisol or ACTH, which may result in levels that are "low normal" when tested. Again, no red flag on the lab report sheet. No wonder this condition is unrecognized in women with hormone problems!

Now, if you look at these symptoms again, you'll see that many are the same as for someone with thyroid problems. This is not a coincidence, as cortisol is necessary to convert T4 into T3, the active element. It's no surprise that antibodies to thyroid, adrenal and ovarian tissues are frequently seen together.[30]

Researchers are only now starting to investigate adrenal and thyroid autoimmune problems as part of a new syndrome, called Polyglandular Autoimmune Disorder, Type II. (Type I occurs in children and is extremely rare.) PGA Type II affects adults around age 30 and is characterized by a gradual antibody response to both adrenal and thyroid tissue. Think of it as Addison's Disease marries Hashimoto's Thyroiditis.[31] Unfortunately, few physicians seem to be aware of this condition. It follows that if one doesn't diagnose Addison's disease, one has no need to treat it. So why would physicians fail to investigate a patient's complaints?

Frankly, I feel it has to do with fear. Doctors are uncomfortable with adrenal hormones and lump all steroids into "anabolic" or body building categories. Steroids are powerful hormones that have been prescribed in the past with little knowledge or concern about the subtle nuances between each of the different steroids. Megadoses were doled out to control inflammatory conditions, causing stomach ulcers, osteoporosis and even Cushing's syndrome. As a result, doctors hesitate to identify a condition for which steroid management is the treatment.

All this may change with the introduction of new tests. Antibodies to 21-hydroxylase, an enzyme produced by the adrenal cortex, are positive when adrenal tissue is damaged, as in Addison's disease, and provides an excellent screening test for this condition.[32] This condition can even incite ovarian antibodies as a cause for premature ovarian failure, or early menopause.[33] In this instance, adrenal antibodies to 17-hydroxylase, an enzyme responsible for the production of androgenic or male hormones, are also positive.[34] It's no surprise that 70% percent of those with autoimmune adrenal insufficiency and PGAII are females. Now, there are many more tests that an endocrinologist can order to confirm the diagnosis, so I don't want you to think adrenal antibodies are the definitive answer. However, the presence of antibodies should "raise the flag" for an ACTH stimulation test in order to confirm adrenal insufficiency.[30] So how do you treat this condition?

It only takes a little bit of hydrocortisone a day to make a world of difference to those with primary or secondary adrenal failure. However, like many things in medicine, how much and when to take it is debatable. The consensus seems to be 15 to 20 mg of Cortef (hydrocortisone) a day is enough to replicate the normal amount produced by the adrenals under non-stressful conditions. Some recommend equally divided doses at 5mg a day, while others feel 10mg in the AM with 5mg around 4PM is best. I have even seen support for once a day dosing. However, hydrocortisone is a short acting drug that often fails to mimic the normal daily rhythm of cortisol. This can result in complaints of fatigue, headache and nausea in the morning. For this reason, some endocrinologists prefer Prednisone (deltacortisone), which takes much longer before it is completely metabolized in the body. Prednisone is often given at 5mg in the morning, followed by an afternoon dose of 5mg Cortef for those who have a more rapid metabolism. In some instances, taking Prednisone at bedtime is preferred, as it has a greater effect at lowering the ACTH response that occurs around 4 AM. Since cortisol secretion normally increases under stress, illness, altitude changes (such as flying), or extremes in temperature, anyone on therapy should increase their medication temporarily to avoid an adrenal crisis. Treatment of the mineralcorticoid deficiency that results in low blood pressure and salt cravings can be handled by taking Florinef (9a-fluoro-hydrocortisone) in a usual dose of .1mg daily.

Adrenal problems are one of extremes — either too little or too much cortisol. So how do you know if your adrenal gland is becoming an overachiever?

YOU MIGHT HAVE AN OVERACTIVE ADRENAL GLAND IF (CUSHING'S DISEASE)

- You're so fat little children try to push you back into the ocean
- Strange dark purplish stretch marks appear on your thighs, stomach or bra line
- Your face is so ruddy you could play Mrs Claus without the makeup
- Your sex drive...what sex drive?
- You can't get to sleep, but when you do, you wake up at 2AM unable to fall asleep again until after 5AM
- Your eighty-year-old mother has better muscle tone than you do
- You get offered the role of Igor now that a strange hump has grown on the back of your neck
- You're too young for menopause but you no longer menstruate
- Your face is so round cows try jumping over it
- You need to pluck your chins hairs on a daily basis
- You've got acne like a teenager
- Your blood pressure is higher than Ally McBeal's skirts
- You feel depressed, irritable and can't concentrate

If you answered yes to six or more of these symptoms, you may be experiencing adrenal hyperplasia, or Cushing's syndrome. This syndrome is caused by excessive cortisol production. Like Addison's disease, it is more common in women especially between the ages of 25-40. A more specific problem, called Cushing's Disease, is caused by benign tumors located in the adrenal glands or in the anterior lobe of the pituitary. In either the disease or the syndrome, women experience a sudden weight gain that causes purple striations or stretch marks, on their thighs, stomach and under their arms. Insulin resistance causes elevated glucose levels which lead to diabetes.

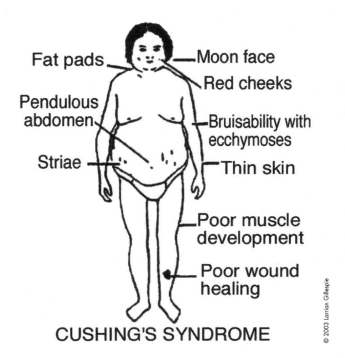

© 2003 Larrian Gillespie

Figure 10 **Appearance of a woman with Cushings Syndrome**

Brenda's story

During my thirties, I began to grow a tiny little mustache, and some chin hair. I noticed I felt fatigued more but all of this was very subtle and did not send me running to the doctor. Over the next few years I noticed purple stretch marks appearing on my hips and I now had a Buddha Belly. My hair was coarse and my skin was so rough and dry I had a red face. I started to gain weight. I had killer PMS symptoms, all of which got much worse over a year or so. When I went to the gynecologist I brought a picture of my former self. My cholesterol was over 300 and I was referred to an endocrinologist.

The endo peered at my stretch marks, uttered "Cushings" and left the room. I have never seen him since. I have had to fight to get the proper tests and to see qualified doctors. It has been a nightmare. I'm not the frightened pushover I was when I started out. It amazes me how many symptoms are blamed on "obesity." This is why I make a point of detailing that my foot problems, hirsutism, virtually everything came BEFORE the weight gain. Fat was one of the very last symptoms to show up.

Now you would think all these symptoms would make any elevator operator push the Cushinoid button, but many doctors fail to investigate these complaints, writing them off as stress, an overactive fork, or menopause. Women who suffer from too much cortisol production in their body have a 55% chance of having a primary thyroid condition, such as Hashimoto's thyroiditis.[35] So what is the best screening test for Cushing's?

It's so simple one could spit...literally! Cortisol is the ONLY hormone that remains stable in saliva for at least 24 hours. This makes it an ideal medium to use for painless screening. Salivary samples are best taken at 8AM and 8PM. The setup is simple. First, rinse your mouth but DO NOT brush your teeth. Now think about a juicy steak and feel your mouth fill up with saliva. Spit into a clean cup, then pour the contents into the transport tube. If you are going to mail the specimen, it would be best to freeze it overnight and let the postal service do the thawing.

Normal values for women at 8 AM are 9.8 ± 3.1 mmol/l with a range between 4.8 – 18 mmol/l. Evening levels should be around 3.9± 0.2 mmol/l with a range between 2.2 – 4.2 mmol/l.

An elevated salivary cortisol test, done at bedtime, easily confirms the diagnosis.[36] Like Addison's, there are numerous other tests, which assist the physician in locating the site of the problem. Looking for an elevated prolactin level, a hormone produced by the pituitary gland, can screen for pituitary lesions. An MRI of the adrenal glands and pituitary should visualize any adenomas in the tissue. The treatment of Cushing's disease usually requires removal of the active hormone secreting tumor.

Now that you understand the function of your adrenal glands, let's move on to the stuff that makes us women — our ovaries.

Disease	Cortisol	ACTH
Cushing's disease (pituitary tumor making ACTH)	High	High
Adrenal tumor	High	Low
"Ectopic" ACTH (ACTH made by a tumor outside the pituitary, usually in the lung)	High	High
Addison's disease (adrenal damage)	Low	High
Hypopituitarism	Low	Low

Figure 14 **Summary of Adrenal Problems**

OVARIAN PROBLEMS

It's true that good things come in small packages – even your ovaries. Barely larger than a small chicken egg, each ovary contains approximately 500,000 eggs at birth. During puberty, some of these eggs begin to move toward the center of the ovary, forming follicles, or "ovums in training." Once the pituitary/ hypothalamus team sends out the appropriate amounts of leutenizing hormone, an ovum is selected for "ovulation." If fertilization occurs in the fallopian tube, the egg implants into the wall of the uterus and starts the development of a fetus. No fertilization? The egg is discarded and with it the preliminary uterine lining. This shedding is called a menstrual period.

Summary of the Menstrual Cycle

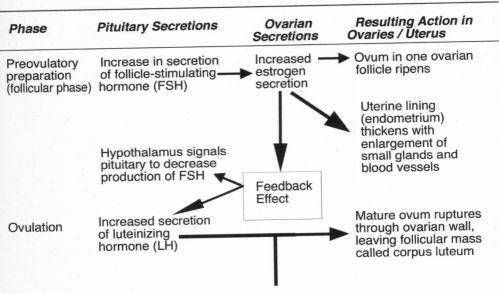

Phase	Pituitary Secretions	Ovarian Secretions	Resulting Action in Ovaries / Uterus
Preovulatory preparation (follicular phase)	Increase in secretion of follicle-stimulating hormone (FSH)	Increased estrogen secretion	Ovum in one ovarian follicle ripens
			Uterine lining (endometrium) thickens with enlargement of small glands and blood vessels
	Hypothalamus signals pituitary to decrease production of FSH	Feedback Effect	
Ovulation	Increased secretion of luteinizing hormone (LH)		Mature ovum ruptures through ovarian wall, leaving follicular mass called corpus luteum

© 2003 Larrian Gillespie

Figure 11A **Hormonal influence on the menstrual cycle**

Summary of the Menstrual Cycle

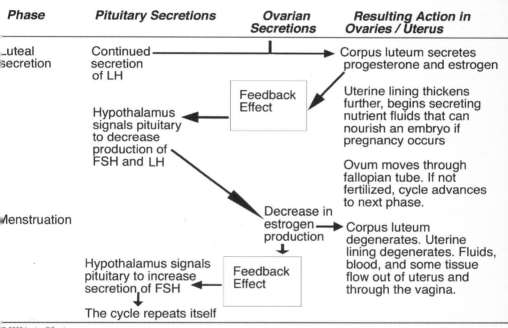

Phase	Pituitary Secretions	Ovarian Secretions	Resulting Action in Ovaries / Uterus
Luteal secretion	Continued secretion of LH		Corpus luteum secretes progesterone and estrogen
		Feedback Effect	Uterine lining thickens further, begins secreting nutrient fluids that can nourish an embryo if pregnancy occurs
	Hypothalamus signals pituitary to decrease production of FSH and LH		Ovum moves through fallopian tube. If not fertilized, cycle advances to next phase.
Menstruation		Decrease in estrogen production	Corpus luteum degenerates. Uterine lining degenerates. Fluids, blood, and some tissue flow out of uterus and through the vagina.
	Hypothalamus signals pituitary to increase secretion of FSH	Feedback Effect	
	The cycle repeats itself		

Figure 11B **Hormonal influence on the menstrual cycle**

HORMONE LEVELS

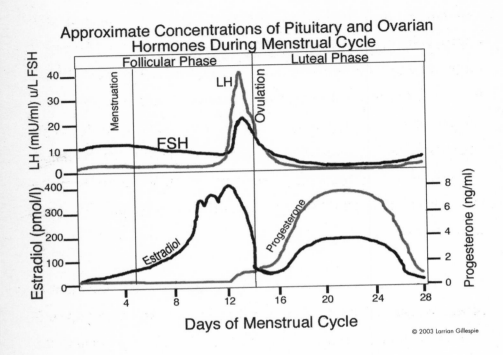

Figure 12 **Concentrations of hormones during a normal cycle**

A concert of hormones plays about during your menstrual cycle, with each one taking the lead at a particular moment. This can cause mass confusion, however, when it comes to the appropriate time to "test" your hormones. So why would doctors commonly order studies on day 3 of your menstrual cycle? Blame it on in vitro fertilization protocols, which need your hormone levels tested on day 3 (the quiet phase) in order to begin pharmaceutical stimulation of ovulation. If you are trying to investigate the normal cycle, however, each hormone requires evaluation on a different day in order to determine its peak performance.

Day 1 of your menstrual cycle is the first day you start to bleed. Normal bleeding is usually 4 days, but can extend up to 5-7 days in some women. This part of the cycle is called the follicular phase. All the hormones are playing quietly in the background. By day 5, estradiol has started to rise above the crowd, taking the lead until day 10. Estradiol levels start to drop just as Leutenizing (LH) and Follicle Stimulating hormone (FSH) peak, in order to induce ovulation somewhere around days 12-14. This completes the follicular phase. The luteal phase is where all the hormonal trouble begins. If you have not ovulated, there is no corpus luteum to produce progesterone, whose purpose is to thicken the uterine lining in preparation for receiving the ovum. If ovulation has occurred, leaving the corpus luteum or collapsed

Salivary vs Serum Results

Saliva testing has become popular, seeming like a natural alternative for those of us who are "needle phobic." Unfortunately, it has also become the "standard" for those health practitioners unable to order any studies that require "piercing the skin." When a study was done comparing saliva testing using cotton swabs and serum levels, the salivary ones were all wet. Testosterone, DHEA, progesterone and estradiol were artificially high. In contrast, cortisol and DHEA-S were not affected by the material used to collect the sample.[38] So if you want accurate testing of your hormones, stick with the serum values.

follicle behind in the ovary, progesterone levels will peak around day 21.

TEST WITH A PURPOSE IN MIND

As you can see, it depends on what kind of hormonal problem you are encountering that determines **when** is the best time to test a particular hormone. If you are trying to get pregnant, testing FSH and estradiol on day 3 is important to determine if someone has an adequate "ovarian reserve" — enough eggs in the bank. A serum FSH between 2-7 on day three reflects excellent "ovarian reserve", meaning you should have lots of good eggs still in your ovaries. A level between 9-24 indicates depleting levels in your egg savings account, and an FSH over 25 says you should check the side of your tampax box for a suicide note from your ovaries.

Estradiol levels are also important on day 3, as a serum value over 80 pmol/l may be artificially lowering an elevated FSH, indicating a less than desirable chance for conception to occur. If you want to know if you have ovulated, you can either use the sialic acid test referred to in Chapter 1 or you can test your progesterone level on day 21. A serum value above 3-6 ng/ml indicates successful ovulation. Remember to fast and have your progesterone level drawn early in the morning, as eating a meal or testing in the afternoon will result in a level **SIGNIFICANTLY** lower.[37]

PREMENSTRUAL SYNDROME (PMS)

Moody? Cranky? Feel like you have a **Puffy Mid Section?** You're not alone, as nearly three quarters of all women will experience a cluster of symptoms known as PMS sometime throughout their menstrual cycle.

YOU MIGHT HAVE PMS IF

- You start looking for your shotgun because all men are stupid
- Your children find you huddled in the closet with chocolate smears on your face
- You wear pie plate bras to protect your sensitive, swollen breasts
- You weep at the sight of baby animals, your teenager's haircut or the price of avocados in the store
- You feel so tired you can't keep your eyes open

• You feel overwhelmed, depressed
• String-draw pants become your new daily uniform

If you answered yes to four or more of these symptoms, you may suffer from premenstrual syndrome. So how do you find out the cause for this condition?

Important hormone information is contained in your Day 3 FSH and day 14 estradiol levels. An estradiol that does not exceed 200 pmol/l indicates you are not producing enough estradiol during ovulation, which results in changes in the ratio of progesterone to estradiol in the second half of your cycle. PMS is really about the erratic swings in estradiol production, which can be caused by stress, aging, high glycemic carbohydrates and lack of exercise. So what can help treat PMS once you control the factors I listed?

Just a splash of estradiol. Using as little as .25mg estradiol on days 10-14 can calm down abnormal signals from the hypothalamus, resulting in smooth sailing for the second half of your cycle.

And don't forget your thyroid if PMS is bugging your life. Swings in estradiol can alter thyroid-binding globulin, affecting how much thyroxine is available for use by your tissue.[39, 40, 41] Changes in your TSH levels can increase your sensitivity to salt, causing one to blow up like a puffer fish in a whistling contest. Diet is another critical factor in PMS management. By consuming low glycemic carbohydrates high in tryptophan, and adequate protein sources, you can increase the production of serotonin, a mood-stabilizing hormone.[42] (see Table 7) Don't forget to include pyridoxal-5-phosphate, a post-liver metabolized form of B6, to complete the metabolism of tryptophan into serotonin. Women lose twice as much pyridoxal-5-phosphate in their urine as men, which may explain our tendency towards depression.[43] Enteric coated tablets (this means they will only dissolve in your small intestine and not in your stomach) in the 20mg range are sufficient for most women.

LOW GLYCEMIC CARBOHYDRATES HIGH IN TRYPTOPHAN	
Tofu	Roasted Pumpkin Seeds
Most Soy products	Gluten flour
Black-eyed Peas	yogurt
Black and English Walnuts	beans
Almonds	2% milk
Sesame Seeds	

PROTEIN SOURCES HIGH IN TRYPTOPHAN	
Meat	cheddar
turkey	Gruyere
fish	Swiss cheese
tofu	eggs

Table 7 **Sources high in tryptophan**

POLYCYSTIC OVARIAN SYNDROME

Pity the fat, bearded lady in the circus who didn't have a decent gynecologist! Polycystic ovarian syndrome, or PCOS, affects 5% to 10% of women, making it the most common hormone disorder for women in their reproductive years. It has multiple causes which can result in facial and body hair growth, acne, weight gain, insulin resistance, and absent or missed menstrual periods. More importantly, if left undiagnosed and untreated, it can lead to diabetes, high blood pressure, heart disease, and an increased risk of endometrial and ovarian cancer.[44]

YOU MIGHT SUFFER FROM PCOS IF

- You have a family history of infertility or irregular periods
- You are of Hispanic descent
- Your first period started before the age of eleven
- You have been treated with antidepressants, anti-seizure medication for long periods at a time
- You've acquired a spider body...thin arms and legs and a Buddha Belly
- You've started losing hair just like a man
- You thought you might be in menopause because you haven't had a period in a long time
- You've developed guerrilla hair growth around your mouth, back, nipples, and chest, along with acne
- Your sex drive...again...what sex drive?

If you answered yes to seven or more of these symptoms, you may have PCOS. Unfortunately, not all women have a majority of the signs or symptoms of this condition. Thin women may have PCOS and no facial hair growth. You can be overweight and not suffer from PCOS. All the symptoms listed in this profile can be caused by either ovarian, adrenal or pituitary changes that increase the amount of circulating testosterone in the body.[45, 46]

The "cardinal" features of PCOS are excess hair growth and menstrual irregularity from a failure to ovulate. So how do you know if you've ovulated? Do not confuse having a period as "proof" of ovulation, as shedding can occur as a result of anovulatory changes in the ratio of progesterone to estradiol. Don't believe me? Just look at what happens on birth control pills. No ovulation — yet you get a period at 28 days. So, the only proof of ovulation is a serum progesterone level drawn on day 21. However, the sialic acid tester is a reasonable "first" screening approach if you are suspicious you are not ovulating.

Since changes in testosterone can come from several sources, how do you know if your ovaries are acting a little "butch?" An ultrasound of the ovaries, demonstrating the "ring of cysts," is a hallmark of this condition[47].

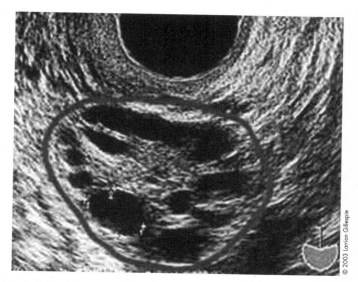

© 2003 Larrian Gillespie

Figure 13 **Hypoechogenic (dark lucent circles) ring of follicles or cysts around the outer edge of the ovary indicate anovulation consistent with PCOS**

All women with PCOS have an increased sensitivity to androgens, or male hormones produced by our bodies. The three major circulating androgens are:

- Androstenedione (of which 90% is produced in the ovaries)
- DHEA-S (mainly produced in the adrenal glands)
- Testosterone (produced from the ovaries and adrenal glands in equal amounts)

When your body produces too much androstenedione, it is converted to estrone, which is stored in body fat. Estrone has a stimulating effect on leutenizing hormone (LH), while suppressing follicle stimulating hormone (FSH). When the LH/FSH ratio is elevated, more androstenedione is produced by the ovary but not converted into estrone, which keeps the cycle of LH production going. Some of that excess androstenedione is converted into testosterone. Estradiol levels may be low to normal, with estrone levels increased due to the enzymes in fat, called aromatase, converting androstenedione into estrone.

The pituitary gets into the act by releasing large amounts of prolactin, which stimulates the adrenals to produce DHEA-S and cortisol. Stress can increase cortisol and DHEA-S production, which perpetuates the abnormal LH/FSH response. Insulin levels rise and change your ovaries' response to LH. Now an entire cascade of events happens, which results in decreased sex hormone binding globulin (SHBG), allowing more androgens to circulate and beat up your tissue, causing acne, manly hair growth in feminine areas and thinning hair.

LATE ONSET CONGENITAL ADRENAL HYPERPLASIA

There is another condition that presents with polycystic ovaries, called late onset congenital adrenal hyperplasia, or LOCAH. This disorder, once thought rare, is due to a deficiency in cortisol, causing the adrenals to overcompensate by making too much testosterone and DHEA. Women commonly complain of acne, excess facial hair growth and menstrual problems, such as infertility. Several adrenal enzymes may be lacking, such as 21, 17, and 11 hydroxylases, which can result in anxiety and epileptic seizures.[101,102] An ACTH stimulation test is the best screening test for this condition.

Insulin Resistance by a Neck

In a fascinating study, researchers found the circumference of your neck to be associated with the following risks of developing the metabolic syndrome, PCOS and insulin resistance:

less than 39 cm — low risk

39-42cm — intermediate risk

greater than 42 cm — high risk

Weight loss resulted in lower androgen and insulin levels, in addition to wearing a smaller necklace size.[48]

So what laboratory tests should your doctor order to be certain this condition is not missed?

- Prolactin
- Estrone
- Testosterone
- DHEA-S
- Corticotropin-stimulated 17-alpha hydroxyprogesterone
- Fasting blood glucose
- Insulin level
- Pelvic transvaginal ultrasound

No two women with PCOS have the EXACT same metabolic problems, so treatment needs to be tailored to their specific profile. Since all women with PCOS have a hypersensitivity to androgens, the following medications may be useful:

- Weight loss is the first treatment, as it can result in lowered insulin and testosterone levels along with improved

Hair Loss, Unwanted Hair Growth in Women

Until recently, hair loss in women was not "categorized" as it is in men. However, this is changing as more interest in treating female hair loss develops. Traditionally, women were thought to lose hair in a generalized "thinning" pattern on the crown or top of the head. However, the hairline did not recede.

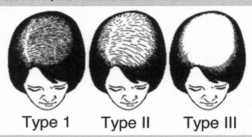

Type 1   Type II   Type III

© 2003 Lorrain Gillespie

Figure 14 **Hair loss patterns in women**

Unfortunately, this neglected the temporal balding pattern seen with thyroid/adrenal issues, where bald points develop at the temples and behind the ears, while leaving the center hairline intact. Researchers are now linking elevated free testosterone levels with this pattern.

Most women complain of "thinning" hair, or excessive hair shedding. This condition, called telogen effluvium, can be caused by diet deficiencies, in particular iron (low serum ferritin levels); crash dieting, thyroid problems, extreme stress (both emotional and physical), high fevers, drugs such as propanolol, Vitamin A excess and anticoagulants; estrogen changes and sudden blood loss.[49]

Unwanted hair growth in a male pattern, called hirsutism, is one of the most psychologically devastating conditions women face with abnormal hormone production. Excess testosterone is the key trigger, but increased body fat and hyperinsulinemia can increase the sensitivity of hair follicles to testosterone.

Saw palmetto, or finasteride, the active ingredient in Propecia and Proscar can help block the effect of DHT, an enzyme that sensitizes hair follicles to testosterone. [50] A new topical cream, Vaniqa, contains eflornithine, which blocks ornithine decarboxylase in skin, preventing hair regrowth.

estradiol/progesterone values. An ideal book on this subject for women facing hormone problems is The Goddess Diet Book, which I wrote to explain how to choose foods that harmonize with your hormones. You will find information on this book in Chapter 9.

• Spironolactone acts by blocking the androgen receptor from "seeing" DHT. It may also suppress 17/20-hydroxylase activity, blocking androgen production. It has minimal effect on free testosterone and androstenedione. Although it can reduce unwanted sexual hair growth or hirsutism, it has no effect on hair regrowth.[51] Usual dosage is 50 to 100mg per day in divided doses.

• Birth control pills containing anti-androgens, such as Yasmin, reduce androgen production by blocking ovulation. They can also increase SHBG, which lowers the amount of free circulating testosterone. The newer pills contain progestins such as dosgestrel, norgestimate and ethynodiol diacetate, which have less androgenic properties to them.

• Finasteride (Propecia) is as effective as spironolactone at blocking DHT binding. The usual dose is 1mg.

• Bromocriptine (Parlodel) is useful in women with elevated prolactin levels. It helps to re-establish ovulation and cycling in women with PCOS.[52] The usual dose is 2.5-15 mg a day, taken at night.

• Steroids, such as Prednisone, are helpful if birth control pills and spironolactone fail to suppress DHEA-S or testosterone adequately. A dose of 2.5 to 5mg should be taken at night to blunt corticotropin stimulation of the adrenal gland the following morning.[53]

• Metformin, an oral insulin drug, increases muscle glucose uptake, which lowers serum insulin levels. It raises SHBG and lowers testosterone much like birth control pills. Women treated in this manner spontaneously ovulated, even without losing weight. The recommended dosage is between 1,500 to 2,000 mg per day.

• Estradiol may be given to women with low estradiol levels in order to assist in ovulation. The usual dose is .25mg Estrace orally.

OVARIAN CYSTS

One of the most common signs of a hormone problem is the formation of an ovarian cyst. When ovulation fails to occur normally, the egg may become trapped in its casing, which continues to fill with hormone-rich fluid. This stretches the ovary like a balloon. Called follicular cysts, these become more common as one nears menopause. Thyroid problems can also cause ovulatory disturbances. Fortunately, the majority of cysts are not cancerous.

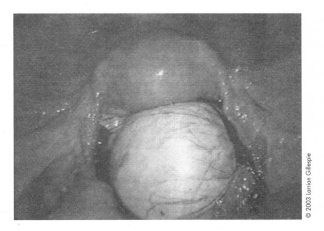

© 2003 Larrian Gillespie

Figure 15 **Large ovarian cyst behind the uterus.
It is filled with straw colored fluid produced by the ovary**

An ultrasound is the best test to "see" a cyst. If it contains fluid only, seen as a clear echo, it is considered benign. If jagged edges or mixed shadows are seen within the cyst, it raises the suspicion this could be a tumor or an endometrioma.

ENDOMETRIOSIS

Endometriosis is a condition in which cells from the endometrium, or lining of the uterus, are found outside the organ. Implants may be located along sensory nerve pathways in the pelvis or within the ovary and fallopian tubes. In many cases, endometrial implants invade the bowel, bladder, diaphragm, or hide under the ureters. No two cases are ever alike.

Women with endometriosis represent various failures in the ovulation mechanism. Some women simply don't ovulate, resulting in low progesterone levels. Some produce inadequate levels of progesterone, called a luteal phase defect. Women who

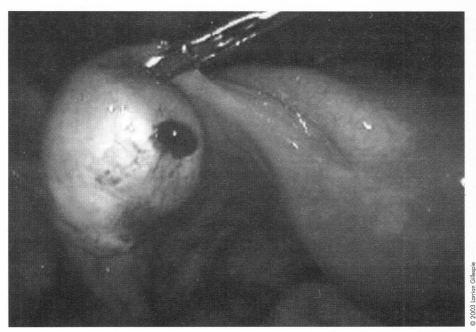

Figure 16 **The black spot is an endometrial implant on the ovary**

fail to rupture the follicle leak fluid into the pelvis, which allows endometrial cells to survive and grow without the "killing" effect of progesterone. In short, ovulation defects cause endometriosis.

New evidence supports the theory that endometriosis represents another "autoimmune" disorder, much like hypothyroidism. In fact, women with endometriosis have a much higher incidence of Hashimoto's thyroiditis, and collagen-vascular disorders such as rheumatoid arthritis and lupus.[54, 55]

YOU MIGHT HAVE ENDOMETRIOSIS IF

- You suffer from severe menstrual cramps
- You experience pelvic pain apart from menses
- You complain of a constant backache during menstruation
- Intercourse is painful deep inside
- Bowel movements cause painful spasms
- You're unusually tired
- You can't tolerate a belt around your waistline
- You never have a normal, daily bowel movement
- When you get your period, it always causes diarrhea
- Exercising or stretching causes abdominal pain
- A pelvic exam at the gynecologist's office puts you in tears
- You can't pass a toilet without feeling the need to urinate
- You have pain before and after, but not DURING urination

If you experience eight or more of these symptoms, you may have endometriosis and should see your doctor.

HOW TO DIAGNOSE ENDOMETRIOSIS

A portion of the ovary may lose its central blood supply, which can result in a cyst filled with blood, called an endometrioma. On ultrasound, it has the appearance of a solid mass, or may show "mixed shadows" which imply a tumor. However, an MRI may be useful in defining those shadows better. In this case, an endometrioma with a dependent clot was diagnosed prior to surgical removal.

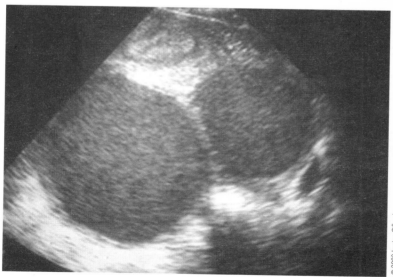

Figure 17 **Ultrasound showing a solid appearing mass attached to the ovary**

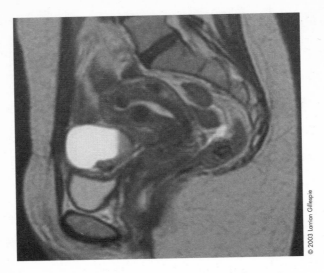

Figure 18 **MRI clarifies this mass is an endometrioma (white spot) with a clot in the base**

TREATMENT OPTIONS

Simple ovarian cysts usually resolve spontaneously within eight weeks (two cycles), but sometimes it's necessary to shut down the system with birth control pills. This short-circuits abnormal hormonal pathways, and helps to establish a normal cycle and prevent further follicular cysts. A repeat ultrasound should be done to confirm your cyst has pulled a "disappearing act." However, if it remains, surgical exploration and removal may be considered.

What if you don't have cycles, such as women in menopause? Follicular cysts may occur in women taking estrogen therapy. However, in my experience, they represent unrecognized endocrine imbalances, such as thyroid disease. So, don't rush into a surgical procedure without requesting thyroid studies. It could prevent you from being on the "cutting edge."

Treatment of endometriosis should be focused on controlling pain, controlling the disease or enhancing fertility. Birth control pills may benefit women in the early stages of this disease by shutting down the normal cycle. More advanced cases, however, may require GnRH analogs (Lupron, Synarel). These affect the hypothalamus and stop ovulation. However, since this process mimics menopause, the addition of estradiol is now recommended.

Progesterone cream may improve fertility issues by "killing" endometrial cells that spill into the pelvic fluid which forms after the egg ruptures. However, it does not CAUSE ovulation to occur. Finally, investigating other autoimmune disorders is warranted in women with endometriosis, as bringing thyroid antibodies under control with adequate therapy and selenium may lower antibodies to the ovaries.

Chemicals that disrupt ovarian function

There is a significant debate about chemicals that mimic, enhance or inhibit estrogen hormones. Some are relating them to an increased incidence of endometriosis, breast cancer, and other hormone-related diseases.[57] Organochlorine pesticides and their metabolites have been shown to interfere with estrogen metabolism by preventing its natural inactivation, leading to increased levels of estradiol.[58] Contrary to some beliefs, there is no definitive proof that heating food in plastic containers, such as in a microwave, or letting plastic wrap come in contact with fat, can affect your estrogen levels. However, if you have ovarian problems, play safe and only use ceramic or glass containers. Paper towels may be substituted for plastic wrap covers.

OVARIAN CANCER

Although ovarian cancer is rare, I am including it in this workbook because it takes a woman's intuition to find it early enough to cure. Ovarian cancer is a silent disease, with few signs or symptoms before it has spread outside of the ovary. In my medical experience, the few women who were eventually diagnosed with ovarian cancer "intuitively" knew something was wrong, but were dismissed as "anxious women" by their doctors.

If you look at the list of symptoms below, you will see they are similar to those of endometriosis or other hormonal problems, so don't panic when you read them!

SIGNS AND SYMPTOMS OF OVARIAN CANCER

- Unexplained change in bowel and/or bladder habits such as constipation urinary frequency, and/or incontinence
- Gastrointestinal upset such as gas, indigestion, and/or nausea
- Unexplained weight loss or weight gain
- Pelvic and/or abdominal pain or discomfort
- Pelvic and/or abdominal bloating or swelling
- A constant feeling of fullness
- Fatigue
- Abnormal or postmenopausal bleeding
- Pain during intercourse

A transvaginal ultrasound is the first step if you suspect something is not "right" with your ovaries. This exam is relatively inexpensive and is considered the best screening test for ovarian cancer.[56] However, an MRI allows for better definition of an ovarian mass. The treatment of ovarian cancer is beyond the scope of this workbook, but you will find many excellent resources on the internet.

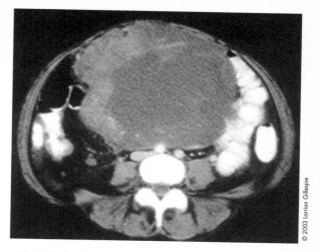

© 2003 Larrian Gillespie

Figure 19 **MRI of a large ovarian cancer filling the abdomen.
Notice it has both dark and light shadows.
Doctor's blamed this woman's expanding waistline on her diet.**

5

MENOPAUSE

Trying to navigate your way through menopause may seem as hopeless as scrubbing a battleship with a Q-tip. Everywhere you turn the news, and even doctors, are stirring a kettle of fear called hormones. So let's step back, grab that cuppa tea or coffee, and carefully evaluate the natural life phase called menopause.

Menopause is a medical term used to describe the time one year AFTER you stop having periods, which occurs around age 51. But the ten or more years before your ovaries go "two claws up" can put you on a hormonal roller-coaster ride every month. So, in this chapter I'm going to separate your approach to management into the pre-menopause phase (those ten or more screwy years) and the post menopause phase (all the rest of your life).

PRE-MENOPAUSE

Let's take a look again at a "normal" menstrual cycle. Estradiol is the major player, peaking levels around day 12. If ovulation has occurred, progesterone takes over the leading role, preparing the uterus for a fertilized egg. If no conception has occurred, both estradiol and progesterone levels plummet and menstruation occurs.

As your reserve of eggs begins to drop, the pituitary gets a change in signals, which shifts the LH response up a few days. This results in a shortened menstrual cycle. If the LH surge fails to rise high enough, anovulation occurs and you have a 36-40 day cycle. This process can vary month to month, making management difficult for most doctor/patient relationships. However, it is NOT impossible, as you will see. So what are the symptoms of perimenopause?

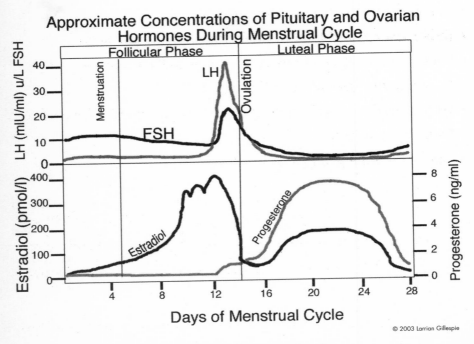

© 2003 Larrian Gillespie

Figure 20 **Normal menstrual cycle**

YOU MIGHT BE PERIMENOPAUSAL IF

- Your moods change faster than a DSL screen
- You applied for sexual amnesty and got it
- You can't concentrate
- You experience menstrual headaches, or begin headaches during your cycle
- You've bought stock in refrigeration companies
- Night sweats have forced you to swim in your bed
- Your vagina chafes
- It's 2AM and you're awake...again.
- Your muscles and joints, especially your thumb, ache
- Everything happens in extremes, especially sweating
- Your bladder doesn't hold enough
- You experience overwhelming depression that turns on and off like a light switch
- PMS stands for pretty much the same

Now you notice these symptoms are basically the same as PMS and menopause, so how are you to know the difference? Here is where listening to your inner "hormone diva" helps out.

As you read in the section on PMS, swings in estradiol, not absolute levels, are responsible for the changes in the menstrual cycle. During perimenopause, your hypothalamus gets "mixed signals" from the ovaries/adrenals/thyroid glands that can impact the release of a follicle. But which tests are the most important?

You will need actually two different sets of tests. FSH levels should be tested on day 3 of your menstrual cycle, as that is when FSH is at its lowest level. An FSH of 25 or above at this time would indicate you are POST menopausal, but anything over 10 would set you in the ballpark of perimenopause. Estradiol should be tested on day 14, as previously mentioned, in order to confirm you are able to achieve a level no less than 200 pg/ml. There is no need to test for progesterone unless one is interested in fertility. Remember, failure to ovulate results in low progesterone levels, and perimenopause is a time of variable ovulation responses.

So, you find yourself in perimenopause. What can you do about it? Some things are simply "out of our control" but there are several factors you CAN change, which will smooth out this time period:

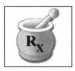

• Diet and exercise

The metabolism of estrogen is very sensitive to the amount of carbohydrate vs. protein in your diet. If you focus on a diet which emphasizes slightly more protein than carbohydrate, you will shift the breakdown of estrogen into a non-estrogenic metabolite that is dumped out in urine.[59] This is a good thing, as it prevents estrogen receptors in your tissue from being overstimulated, which can cause cancer.

This will prevent "estrogen dominance," in which estradiol receptors continue to be stimulated by even more potent estrogen metabolites. Frankly, diets stink, but lifestyle changes can make a significant difference in your health. Exercise can be the missing ingredient in the recipe for a more stable hormone balance. The key is to find an exercise you can "stick" with over time, not just for a few weeks. For an in-depth explanation of how diet and exercise impacts the metabolism of your hormones, please see either "The Menopause Diet" or "The Goddess Diet" books.

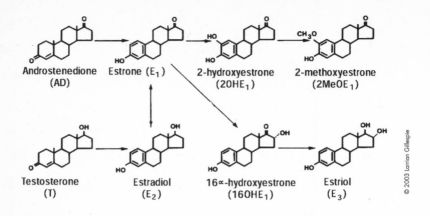

Figure 21 **Metabolic pathways of estradiol**

• Thyroid changes

During perimenopause, women may develop changes in their thyroid function. Unless you bring it to the attention of your doctor, most will ignore this possibility. Remember, lab standards are out of date, so never accept "your values are normal" without obtaining a copy of your lab work and verifying your TSH is between .8 — 1.5 and your thyroid antibodies are negative.

•Adrenal changes

Once estradiol levels start to shift downward, the adrenal gland may react to the stress in our bodies by putting out more cortisol. But in many instances, modified adrenal insufficiency can occur. If you have one autoimmune disorder, such as thyroid disease, you are at an increased risk for developing a second autoimmune condition.[60] Again, failure to consider the diagnosis goes hand in hand with ignoring symptoms that would lead to ordering tests to confirm the diagnosis. For treatment of the above conditions, please refer back to the chapters on each gland.

• Ferritin levels

Changes in your menstrual flow may result in excessive iron loss. Ferritin is the iron carrier molecule that helps to store iron in your body. Chronic inflammatory conditions, such as hypothyroidism or Lupus, will deplete ferritin. Low ferritin levels will also affect your thyroid medication levels, causing women to feel "hyper," especially if they are taking any T3. [14, 61, 62] Maintaining a serum ferritin level around 100ng/ml helps to regulate insulin sensitivity, thyroid, and adrenal function.

•Hormone therapy

Now remove those hands covering your eyes or ears and listen to me. Hormones are not dirty words, and using a splash of the right ones, at the right time can make an enormous difference in your health. In "The Menopause Diet" I have an extensive chapter on this topic, which is also available online from the website, so I won't go into ALL the references and details here. Instead, let me summarize what every hormone diva needs to understand:

• All estrogens are not created equal. Estrone, estriol and 17 beta-estradiol are the NATURAL estrogens in the body that provide various beneficial activity. Synthetic estrogens use words like valerate, esterified, conjugated, ethinyl, estropipate, and norethidrone. The Women's Health Initiative Study focused only on conjugated estrogens and progestins — all synthetic.[63] These hormones increase insulin resistance and incite inflammatory reactions in the body due to their "unnatural" composition. In addition, there was no blood level monitoring of the medication.

• You don't want to "marinate" in hormones when a little "basting" will give you the maximum benefits with the least risk factors. Research shows that a blood level of estradiol between 60-114 pg/ml is sufficient for any postmenopausal woman's needs.[64]

• In the perimenopause phase, a midcycle estradiol should measure over 200 pg/ml in order to provide an even coast downhill during the last 14 days of your cycle. In order to "boost" a limping estradiol level, .5mg of 17 beta-estradiol on days 10-14 may be sufficient to stimulate the LH surge, rather than suppresses it. However, as the duration of perimenopause continues, women may need low dose estradiol support daily. In those situations, .25mg daily is enough to prevent hormone lows.

• Birth control pills should be a last resort. They contain synthetic estrogens and progestins which cause bone resorption, alter hormones in your pituitary and don't contain enough estradiol to prevent these problems.[65] The newer versions, such as Activella, which contains 1mg of estradiol, were designed for post-menopausal women, as no studies have been done to confirm the higher dose of estradiol with the progestin prevents pregnancy.

MENOPAUSE MYTHS

Nothing can set me off on a rant than the numerous myths and attitudes about menopause. Not only do they set my teeth grinding, but I've been known to "bonk" my computer screen over and over when faced with "vampire" tales. Let's see if I can kill them for you!

"I've read women are estrogen dominant during menopause and need progesterone."

How this one got started is a prime example of misrepresenting biochemistry and physiology. Menopause is a time of estrogen LOSS, which results in changes in ovulation. If you don't ovulate, your progesterone level remains low. So, during perimenopause, the ratio of estradiol to progesterone changes in favor of progesterone, NOT estradiol.

"Saliva testing shows I'm estrogen dominant and don't have enough progesterone."

Saliva testing is invalid for all hormones EXCEPT cortisol for numerous reasons: The swab material binds to the hormones and gives false readings by as much as 37% in either direction.[66] Some hormones are simply not stable in saliva and deteriorate quickly. Progesterone is especially tricky, as consuming a meal or testing in the afternoon results in falsely lowered values.[37] No wonder women and their health practitioners have been led down the "estrogen dominant" pathway.

"I'm using a compounded cream with natural estrogen."

This sets my teeth chattering just at the thought of the misrepresentation. Estradiol must be in an alcohol gel form in order to get any absorption across skin. It can be used in a fatty cream form if you are using it on a mucous membrane, such as the vagina, but a cream will NOT let any of the estrogens cross the skin on your arms, stomach, thighs, buttocks, etc. When it comes to "natural" estrogens, women are being told estradiol (20%) and estriol (80%) (sold as a biest cream) are the best choice. Again, no alcohol...no uptake...no blood value changes. Any time I have challenged someone on these compounded or over-the-counter products to a blood estradiol level, it has come back unchanged. Remember, estriol is actually more potent in its effects because it attaches to the same estradiol receptor, increasing the amount of available circulating estradiol, which can cause breast and endometrial cancer.[67, 68] However, since it can't be absorbed in a cream form, no harm, no foul. Taking it orally, however, is a different story. Estriol can induce endometrial hyperplasia just like excessive estradiol.[69,70] It offers no protection against breast cancer and may be associated with a higher risk.[71] All oral preparations of "triest" preparations result in the same estrone and estradiol levels as commercially available estrogens.[72] If you should choose, however, to use these products, you need the same blood level monitoring as anyone taking estradiol. Remember — a blood level between 60-114 pg/ml is sufficient to provide you the maximum bone/brain/eye/heart protection with the least risk.

"My doctor recommends progesterone cream because estrogens cause cancer."

On face value, estrogens CAN cause cancer, just like many environmental chemicals we're exposed to on a daily basis. To eliminate part of the problem of this myth, we are going to exclude all synthetic estrogens and progestins from the discussion. Unlike estradiol, progesterone is fat-soluble and CAN be mixed in a cream format. However, testing of the creams has shown as little as 200mg in total, to as much as 500mg/ml, some with medroxyprogesterone (Provera) mixed in one container.[73] This means women may be getting only a serum increase of 3mg of progesterone a day, instead of the usual 30-50 mg produced by an ovum. Progesterone increases androgenic steroids, such as androstendione, aldosterone and cortisol, which can improve menopausal symptoms.

Oral micronized progesterone has been used in Europe as

part of hormone management therapy. Research done in 1993 erroneously used a technique which measured all the metabolites as progesterone, leading doctors to believe micronized progesterone overcame the metabolism problems.[74] However, it is rapidly metabolized in the liver and has little effect on endometrial hyperplasia.[75,76] The PEPI study used 300mg of micronized progesterone (100mg AM/200mg PM) in order to offset the short half life of oral progesterone.[77] In such high doses, the endometrium became non-reactive after six months. Yet, many women can't tolerate that high an oral dose of progesterone.

Vaginal progesterone, as a gel or suppository, increases receptor sites in the endometrium and is the best method for preventing endometrial hyperplasia.[78] Current recommendations are for 4% progesterone gel applied for four consecutive nights along with transdermal estradiol.

"My doctor says natural progesterone prevents osteoporosis."

In a letter (translation: This is not a peer review research article) to the editors of Lancet, a physician cited a 14% improvement in bone mineral density in the lumbar spine for women using progesterone cream.[79] No controls were used in this study and subsequent, peer-reviewed studies showed NO benefit.[80] However, this has not stopped physicians from mistaking studies using progestins or testosterone derivatives as being synonymous with natural progesterone.[81, 82]

"Japanese women don't complain of menopausal symptoms because they eat soy."

Most Japanese gynecologists are men and the Asian culture has an issue with losing face, especially if one complains. Women suffer in silence rather than confront their male physicians with symptoms that could be treated. Picture the typical elderly Asian woman. You don't visualize someone standing tall and straight, but rather a shrunken, bent over image comes to mind. In a recent study, women in Hong Kong were able to define "menopause," but were unaware the problems of osteoporosis, heart disease, or Alzheimers were associated with it. More significantly, only 8% of these same women were aware hormone therapy could treat these conditions.[83]

The average amount of soy consumed by Asian women contains no more than 40 mg of isoflavones. They do not consume mass quantities of soy products, contrary to popular marketing.[84] In addition, the Asian populace has a completely different liver enzyme profile from Caucasians, making it more difficult for them to break down some medications. So, you can't compare apples and oranges even if they are fruit, when it comes to menopause.

AVAILABLE HORMONE THERAPIES

There is a glut of available hormones in different formats on today's market. Each, however, serves a different purpose.

Product	Description	Availability
Oral products	**SYNTHETIC**	
Premarin	Conjugated estrogens (50-65% estrone, 20-35% equilin)	0.3 mg
		0.625 mg
		0.9 mg
		1.25 mg
		2.5 mg
Prempro	Conjugated estrogens and medroxyprogesterone acetate	0.625 mg
		5 mg
Prempro	Conjugated estrogens and medroxyprogesterone acetate	0.625 mg
		2.5 mg

Table 8A **Hormone products**

Product	Description	Availability
Oral products	**SYNTHETIC**	
Premphase	Conjugated estrogens and medroxyprogesterone acetate	0.625 mg conjugated estrogens
		0.625 mg conjugated estrogens and 5 mg medroxyprogesterone acetate (14 tabs)
Cenestin	Synthetic conjugated estrogens	0.625 mg
		0.9 mg
Activella	Estradiol 17 β (natural estradiol)	1 mg
	Norethindrone acetate	0.5 mg
Estratab, Menest	Esterified estrogens (75-85% estrone, 6-15% equilin)	0.3 mg
		0.625 mg
		1.25 mg
		2.5 mg
Estratest H.S.	Esterified estrogens and methyltestosterone	0.625 mg
		1.25 mg
Estratest	Esterified estrogens and methyltestosterone	1.25 mg
		2.5 mg
Estinyl	Ethinyl estradiol	0.02 mg
		0.05 mg
		0.5 mg
Femhrt 1/5	Ethinyl estradiol and norethindrone acetate	5 μg
		1 mg
Mircette	21 days ethinyl estradiol	20 cg
	Desogestrel	150 mcg
	2 days no hormones	
	5 days ethinyl estradiol	10 mcg

Table 8B **Hormone products**

Product	Description	Availability
Oral products	**SYNTHETIC**	
Yasmin	21 days ethinyl estradiol	30 mcg
	Drospirenone	3 mg
Oral products	**NATURAL**	
Ogen, Ortho-Est, generic	Estropipate (piperazine estrone sulfate)	0.625 mg
		0.75 mg
		1.25 mg
		1.5 mg
		2.5 mg
		3 mg
Estrace	Micronized Estradiol 17 b	0.5mg
		1mg
		2 mg
Vaginal Products	**SYNTHETIC**	
Premarin	Cream:0.625 mg conjugated estrogens/g (estrone 50-65%, equilin 20-35%)	42.5 gm tube
Ortho Dienetrol	Cream: 0.01% dienestrol	78 gm.tube
Vaginal Products	**NATURAL**	
Estrace	Cream: 1.0 mg estradiol/g	42.5-g tube
Ogen	Cream: 1.5 mg estropipate/g	45-g tube
Estring	Ring: 2 mg estradiol (0.75 µg/day)	Single pack
Vagifem	Tablet, vaginal: 25 µg estradiol	Card packs of 5 tabs
Transdermal products	**SYNTHETIC**	
Combipatch	Estradiol 0.05mg, 0.14mg norethindrone acetate/24 hr release	Carton 8 systems

Table 8C **Hormone products**

Product	Description	Availability
Transdermal products	**SYNTHETIC**	
Combipatch	Estradiol 0.05mg, 0.25mg norethindrone acetate/24 hr release	Carton 8 systems
Transdermal products	**NATURAL**	
Estraderm	0.05 mg/24-hr release (4 mg total estradiol content)	Calendar packs (8 and 24 systems)
	0.1 mg/24-hr release (8 mg total estradiol content)	Calendar packs (8 and 24 systems)
Alora	0.05 mg/24-hr release (1.5 mg total estradiol content)	Calendar packs (8 and 24 systems)
	0.075 mg/24-hr release (2.3 mg total estradiol content)	Calendar packs (8 and 24 systems)
	0.1 mg/24-hr release (3 mg total estradiol content)	Calendar packs (8 and 24 systems)
Climara	0.025 mg/24-hr release (2 mg total estradiol content)	In 4s
	0.05 mg/24-hr release (3.9 mg total estradiol content)	In 4s
	0.075 mg/24-hr release (5.85 mg total estradiol content)	In 4s
	0.1 mg/24-hr release (7.8 mg total estradiol content)	In 4s
Esclim	0.025 mg/24-hr release (5 mg total estradiol content)	Calendar pack (6 or 8 systems) or carton of 24 systems

Table 8D **Hormone products**

Product	Description	Availability
Transdermal Products	**NATURAL**	
Esclim (cont.)	0.0375 mg/24-hr release (7.5 mg total estradiol content)	Calendar pack (6 or 8 systems) or carton of 24 systems
	0.05 mg/24-hr release (10 mg total estradiol content)	Calendar pack (6 or 8 systems) or carton of 24 systems
	0.075 mg/24-hr release (15 mg total estradiol content)	Calendar pack (6 or 8 systems) or carton of 24 systems
	0.1 mg/24-hr release (20 mg total estradiol content)	Calendar pack (6 or 8 systems) or carton of 24 systems
Oestrogel	Estradiol 17β 60mg/100gm gel	80 gm tube
Vivelle/Vivelle-Dot	0.0375 mg/24-hr release (3.28/0.585 mg total estradiol content)	Calendar pack (8 or 24 [Vivelle only] systems)
	0.05 mg/24-hr release (4.33/0.78 mg total estradiol content)	Calendar pack (8 or 24 [Vivelle only] systems)
	0.075 mg/24-hr release (6.57/1.17 mg total estradiol content)	Calendar pack (8 or 24 [Vivelle only] systems)
	0.1 mg/24-hr release (8.66/1.56 mg total estradiol content)	Calendar pack (8 or 24 [Vivelle only] systems)

Table 8E **Hormone products**

Product	Description	Availability
Progestins	**SYNTHETIC**	
Amen	Medroxyprogesterone acetate	10 mg
Aygestin	Norethindrone acetate	5 mg
Cycrin	Medroxyprogeterone acetate	2.5 mg
		5 mg
		10 mg
Megace	Megestrol acetate	20 mg
		40 mg
		160 mg
Micronor	Norethindrone	0.35 mg
Nor-QD	Norethindrone	0.35 mg
Ovrette	Norgestrel	0.075 mg
Provera	Medroxyprogesterone acetate	2.5 mg
		5 mg
		10 mg
Depo-provera	Medroxyprogesterone acetate injectable	150 mg
Progestins	**NATURAL**	
Prometrium	Micronized oral progesterone	100 mg
		200 mg
	Vaginal suppositories	25 mg
		50 mg
Crinone gel	90 mg progesterone	8% applicator
	45 mg progesterone	4% applicator

*Natural means it must contain only estradiol 17 β, estrone, estriol or progesterone.

Table 8F **Hormone products**

LOW-DOSE AJUSTIVE HORMONE THERAPY

So, which route of administration and type of hormone therapy is the best to use? It's just like choosing a hat. Not all styles suite every woman. Although all women experience the same physiologic change as we go into menopause, our biologic responses — and our need for hormone therapy — varies. The idea of "generic HRT" for women is outdated and should be replaced by "low-dose adjustive hormone therapy," according to Dr. Morris Notelovitz.[85] I couldn't agree more!

I would not recommend using any synthetic estrogen, as it may cause inflammatory reactions in the body. Progestins have been shown to increase the rate of breast cancer, among other conditions, so it should be used only in the context of contraception. That leaves natural estrogens and progesterone. You already know that progesterone has the maximum benefit with the least side effects when used vaginally, which makes that the preferred delivery method.

Estradiol 17β is the desired estrogen for its benefits and metabolic pathways. There is really little use for estrone or estriol products in estrogen replacement therapy. In the premenopause stage, women have more estradiol than estrone, but post menopause, estrone is the dominant hormone. Any

Tip for improving absorption of oral medication

If you suffer from low gastric acid or feel you are not absorbing medication, you might try dissolving it under your tongue. This allows the lymphatics and blood vessels in this area to "pick up" the drug directly into your circulation. You might also consider using digestive enzymes that contain bromelain, papain and betaine hydrochloric acid when taking oral medication. You can confirm absorption by measuring blood levels of your medication.

Steroid	Reproductive Age	Natural Menopause	Surgical Menopause
Estradiol	100-150	10-15	10
Testosterone	400	290	110
Androstenedione	1900	1000	700
DHEA	5000	2000	1800
DHEAS	3,000,000	1,000,000	1,000,000

Table 9 **Mean Steroid Levels in Women (Values Converted to pg/mL)**

transdermal therapy would be a first choice, as it avoids the liver's metabolism of estradiol into estrone. This means you can use less estradiol and still have the same benefits.

Oral therapies are dependent upon the level of gastric acid in the stomach. As women age, gastric acid levels decrease, making it more difficult to break down drugs in pill format. Absorption problems can usually be avoided by using either liquid (oral), transdermal (skin) or transmucosal (under tongue, vaginal) delivery methods.

HOW MUCH IS ENOUGH?

Like all things, too much of anything can be a bad thing, so it's important to follow your blood estradiol levels when using estrogen replacement therapy. Several studies have shown that, for postmenopausal women (again, dead ovaries, no ovulation), a blood estradiol level between 70-114 pg/ml does not induce endometrial hyperplasia, yet offers the benefit of protecting and strengthening our bones, brain, heart, skin, eyes, and teeth.[64] However, we can't always be certain our metabolism stays fine tuned, so using vaginal progesterone for 5 days every three to four months will induce a period IF you have any endometrial response.[86,87]

An endovaginal ultrasound will show the thickness of your uterine lining. The lining may become thickened during a menstrual cycle, achieving levels of up to 10mm. It may also become thickened during periods of anovulation, thyroid problems or elevated blood estradiol levels from hormone therapy. If the blood estradiol is between 70-114 pg/ml the

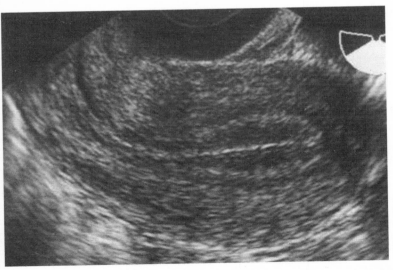

© 2003 Larrian Gillespie

Figure 22 **Normal endometrial thickness. The lighter outline is the full thickness of the uterine lining. It is 2 mm. The white stripe is the endometrial cavity.**

thickness should remain under 6mm. A thickened lining between 6-10mm may indicate endometrial hyperplasia, which is a pre-cancerous condition. Researchers have shown that an endometrial thickness of no more than 5mm is a reliable cut–off range for determining the possible need for an endometrial biopsy.[88]

Now this concept has been around for a few years, yet most doctors are ignorant of the studies AND the safe range for estradiol. As a result, women have been force-fed combination pills with twice as much estrogen as needed, or progestins monthly, making them depressed, fat and increasing their risk for cancer and heart disease. So what can you do if your doctor is "journal challenged" and simply hasn't or won't read these articles? Simply smile and ask for each medication on a separate

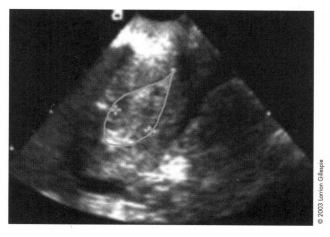

© 2003 Larrian Gillespie

Figure 23 **Ultrasound of uterine lining measuring 10 mm. There are mixed shadows suggestive of possible cancer.**

prescription, then fill only the estradiol. Remember, there are no pharmacy police and a doctor won't know if you take medication "as prescribed" or not. Unfortunately, with today's healthcare system, many women are faced with few choices when it comes to clinicians on their plan, most of whom are forced to tailor their prescriptions to an approved, cost-saving formulary. Your health, however, is YOUR responsibility in the end, as doctors are only advisors.

I can hear you thinking, "But my doctor will be angry with me." Physicians are not your parents! You're an adult with choices and sometimes that means kicking a few doctors off the medical cliff until you find one who listens to YOU. In the end, "Sorry, the drug rep never told me," won't cut it at your funeral if you knowingly allow yourself to endanger your health because of shame.

BREAKTHROUGH BLEEDING

Spotting, whether tiny or bothersome, raises alarm in many women. However, abnormal breakthrough bleeding which occurs for several cycles, or prevents a normal cycle, may indicate fibroids or polyps rather than cancer. Fibroids are steroid dependent benign tumors that respond to either estradiol or progesterone.[89] That means they can grow or regress under the influence of either hormone.

As we've already discussed, changes in your estrogen/thyroid balance can stimulate these same receptors, causing fibroids to either grow or regress. Divas with fibroids should have a complete hormone work-up, including a midcycle estradiol level and thyroid panel. Remember, the lab standards for TSH are incorrect, so be certain your TSH is less than 2 before committing to aggressive surgical therapy, especially a hysterectomy. A reasonable time for balancing hormones is three months. If you still have bleeding despite normal values, ask your doctor if a myomectomy (removing only the fibroid and leaving the uterus intact) or embolization would help.

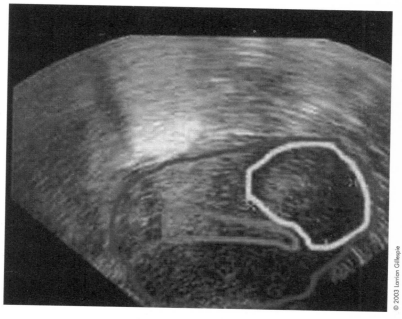

© 2003 Larrian Gillespie

Figure 24 **Ultrasound of uterine fibroid, seen as a ball-like structure attached to the uterine wall.**

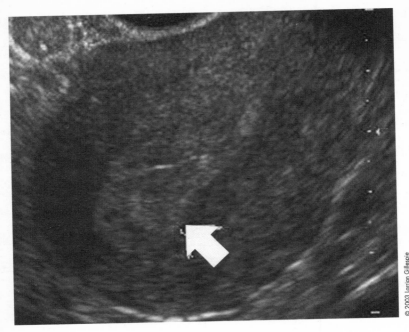

© 2003 Larrian Gillespie

Figure 25 **Uterine polyp seen on ultrasound**

Uterine polyps are another consideration. These little growths of endometrial tissue hang on stalks and irritate the lining of the uterus. They are best seen with a hysteroscopy procedure, where they can be removed and cauterized. If you have very heavy bleeding during your period, polyps along with fibroids should be considered.

THE NON-HORMONAL APPROACH

Not all hormone divas feel comfortable with self-management when it comes to hormone therapy, and some may prefer to try a non-prescription approach. Let's look at how to alleviate the symptoms of menopause — vaginal dryness, hot flashes, mood swings, and sleeping problems.

Vaginal dryness may be the easiest to treat, thanks to many new products that decrease friction between tissues.

Product	Manufacturer	Description	Availability
H-R Lubricating Jelly	Carter-Wallace	Jelly	150 g
Lubricating Jelly	Taro	Jelly	60 g/125 g
K-Y	Johnson and Johnson	Jelly	20 oz/4 oz
K-Y Silk-e Vaginal Moisturizer	Johnson and Johnson (with vitamin E)	Gel	2.4 oz
Lubrin	Kenwood/Bradley	Suppository	5-pack
			12-pack
Maxilube Personal Lubricant	Mission	Gel	90-g tub
			150-g tub
Astroglide	BioFilm	Gel	2.35-oz/5-oz bottle
			5-ml travel packets x 4
Replens	Warner Lambert	Gel	Prefilled, disposable applicators x 8
			35-g tube
Moist Again WHF	Lake	Gel	70.8-g tube
Lubricating Gel	Lake	Gel	4-oz tube

Table 10 **Over-the-Counter Products For Vaginal Dryness**

Hot flashes can respond to protein and arginine, the amino acid found in soybeans, turkey, and chicken. This amino acid helps to increase nitric oxide, a chemical that causes blood vessels to relax. Try using 500mg of arginine a day to stop looking like a furnace. Resveratrol, the ingredient in grape skins and peanuts, acts as an estrogen assistant, binding to the estradiol 17β receptor. Unlike isoflavones in soy, resveratrol does not interfere with thyroid function. Consider trying 100 ug a day to control hot flashes.[90]

Mood swings are a result of changes in the ratio of estradiol to androgenic, or male hormones. Black cohosh (which was the major ingredient in Lydia Pinkham's patented woman's formula) may help smooth things out by lowering LH levels in the brain. Remifemin is a standardized black cohosh preparation available in drugstores.

Sleep disturbances may respond to an herbal combination of Valerian root (Valium was derived from this herb) and Hops, which belongs to the same family of herbs as marijuana in its sedative properties. Several companies manufacture this combination, so check with your local health food store.

PREMATURE MENOPAUSE

You're only 35 yet you're experiencing hot flashes. Could be a case of premature ovarian failure (POF), a condition that affects 1% of women under 40 and is suddenly gaining new attention with the development of 21 hydroxylase antibody testing. Obvious causes, such as radiation therapy or chemotherapy, don't need an explanation, but more women with autoimmune disorders, such as thyroid, are developing this condition.[33, 34] While others have focused on the hypothalamus, new research is pointing to unrecognized adrenal insufficiency triggering anti-ovarian antibodies as the cause.[30, 91, 92]

So how do you know if you might be experiencing premature menopause or POF?

- Irregular periods along with hot flashes
- Vaginal dryness
- Sleep disturbances
- Weight gain
- Changes in body odor (caused by too much progesterone without enough estradiol)
- Headaches
- Mood swings
- Itchy dry skin
- Hair loss
- Electrical shocks or buzzing in your head

As you can see, the symptoms would fit adrenal, thyroid, or ovarian problems. Often women develop POF after a miscarriage, when progesterone levels can suppress immune responses.[93,94] However, in a study of post-delivery hemorrhage, called Sheehan's syndrome, pituitary damage is gradual, setting off a series of autoimmune reactions involving the pituitary that affect adrenal, thyroid and ovarian tissue.[95,96]

Lab studies should include
- FHS done on day 3
- Estradiol done on day 14 (or best guess)
- Progesterone day 21
- 21 hydroxylase antibodies
- prolactin
- thyroid panel (TSH ultrasensitive, Free T3, free T4, thyroid antibodies)

Currently, there is no proven therapy for this condition. However, as one who suffered from it, I can advise you to consider immediate support of your thyroid, adrenal, ovarian, and pituitary hormones. Autoimmune inflammation of the adrenal gland, when caught early, can go into remission and may even prevent the onset of full-blown Addison's disease.[97] Estradiol 1mg plus levothyroxine and low dose cortef should be prescribed as soon as the diagnosis is made.[98] Ironically, a drug used for weight loss, fenfluramine (Pondimen), stimulated LH surges, restoring ovulation. It was withdrawn from the market in 1996.

Now that you have completed "the basics" in understanding your hormones, let's move on to an important issue — negotiating with your doctor.

6

HOW TO NEGOTIATE WITH YOUR DOCTOR

There is probably nothing more important than understanding how to talk so your doctor will LISTEN to you. Most physicians are male. Now think how well your husband or boyfriend listens to you...and he wants sex! So I'm going to help you prepare for a visit and not a confrontation with your healthcare practitioner.

THE RULES OF NEGOTIATION

When faced with a web of tension, such as in a medical office visit, it is important you understand how to use information and power in order to let the doctor have YOUR way. In any negotiation, there are three crucial elements:

1. Information.
2. Time.
3. Power.

As the patient, you assume the doctor has more information about your medical needs than you do. You also believe he has the time to consider various problems, while having the power and authority to make the right decisions about your health. But power is based solely on perception. If you think someone has the power, they have it. If you think you, as the patient, don't have power, even if you do have it — you don't have it! The key to negotiating with a doctor is to attack the problem, NOT the doctor.

I know this sounds simple, but several things can get in the way of a working doctor-patient relationship:

1. Your reaction. When you are under stress and the doctor dismisses your concerns and observations, you naturally feel attacked. The doctor may even shame you into accepting his treatment plan, making you a victim.

2. The doctor's emotion. The doctor/patient relationship is very primal, and much of the behavior that goes on has to do with whether or not the doctor respected his mother. If a doctor is convinced he is right and you are wrong, he merely refuses to listen.

3. The doctor's position. If a doctor is not flexible, he will resort to "sandbox behavior". In his eyes, YOU must give in, because the only other option is for HIM to give in, and he won't do that.

4. Power. The doctor may not see any benefit in reaching a mutually satisfactory relationship. He may fear losing his power by backing down. So, your ideas and suggestions are

rejected for just that reason.

It is unfortunate, but a recent poll of physicians revealed that more than 70% were dissatisfied with medical practice, 25% would no longer consider practicing and 66% would not advise their children to become doctors.[99] Physicians are cranky at the imposition of today's business model on the practice of medicine, which requires them to justify every decision to an authority concerned about cost containment, not the patient's needs. Erosion of authority creates antagonism, and the patient becomes the inadvertent target. It may seem that all medical relationships are doomed, but there are ways to negotiate with your doctor that allows you to maintain a balance of power. It starts with organizing your information.

Believe in Lists

You probably don't go to the grocery store without a shopping list, so why shouldn't the same be true for a visit to a doctor? Physicians have been taught to be wary of patients carrying lists. You can see it in their eyes. They're used to being the one doing the interviewing, and don't react well when faced with a toilet roll's worth of questions. I'll let you in on a secret. Every medical school class is taught to believe that patients carrying lists, especially women, are obsessive individuals who will suck the doctor dry of his time like a medical vampire. However, a family practitioner from Alabama, Dr. John F. Burnum, put a new spin on all this when he wrote, in his article in **The New England Journal of Medicine** that list-writing patients were quite sane.[100]

"Traditional medical wisdom holds that patients who relate their complaints to their physicians from lists are, ipso facto, emotionally ill. DeGowin and DeGowin in their venerable textbook on diagnosis (used by all medical students in their first year) say that note writing is 'almost a sure sign of psychoneurosis. The patient with organic disease does not require references to written notes to give the essence of his story.' But, said Dr. Burnum, "note writing is a normal, honorable practice that can be used to advantage in patient care."

Dr. Burnum decided to observe seventy-two list-writing patients. "Almost all of these emotionally normal list writers had serious physical disorders. Patients with organic disease, therefore, do refer to written notes to give the essence of their story—and not because they are peculiar or crazy."

Note writers simply want to get things straight, he said. Even though they may be anxious and distraught, they are nevertheless seeking clarity, order, information, and control, and trying to avoid wasting the doctor's time.

"Notes may be of great help in the orderly transfer of information to the physician. Medical care turns on communication. Whatever helps patients express themselves and helps physicians understand patients is acceptable."

I agree wholeheartedly with Dr. Burnum. Many list-writing patients do have complicated disorders. It takes time to diagnose such cases, and it requires considerable skill on the part of the physician to interview such patients.

In fact, many physicians do not know how to coax patients into revealing important information—especially small things that the patient may think are inconsequential, but which turn out to reveal aspects of a disease process. In medicine, as in other walks of life, there are few skilled interviewers. So, it's time to sharpen your communication skills.

YOUR HEALTH SCRAPBOOK

First, let's start with creating a health scrapbook. Go to any office supply store and purchase a standard, WHITE binder (black has negative associations and DON'T purchase anything in red, which implies alarm like a "red flag"). Get a 3 hole punch so you can easily file documents into categories in your binder. Pick up a packet of eight separator tabs, a glue stick and a label maker. Neatness counts.

Next, be sure to have plenty of plain white paper for your printer. A typed rather than handwritten history, implies both organization and respect. Remember, you want to give the doctor the impression you are taking your healthcare seriously, just like a business plan. Become familiar with your word processing program, and learn the basics for using a spreadsheet such as Excel or Quatro to organize your medications, observations, or whatever seems to fit a flow sheet concept. What you are doing is creating something that is familiar to your doctor — just like the flow charts at the foot of a patient's bed, which list temperature, blood pressure, urine output, and other important data which need to be analyzed in a sequential manner. Familiarity breeds comfort, and you want to make your doctor comfortable with all the information you have gathered. Remember, the doctor may be the head, but you are the neck that turns that head in any direction!

The FEMALE Formula

Here's what you need to get organized when preparing for a visit to the doctor. Use your powerful "FEMALE" formula. Each letter stands for an important aspect of preparing to establish a successful partnership with your physician:

- Facts
- Evolution
- Medications
- Associated problems
- Laboratory records
- Emotion

Facts

Before you go to the store to spend your money, you sit down and assess what you really need. Do the same preparation for your office visit. What do you need from this physician and how are you going to get it? Do you need an investigator to unravel a mystery, or does the problem seem pretty clear to you? You should be organized when you go, so take an inventory of your complaints and observations. Women are extremely accurate observers of their bodies. Try to keep your thoughts as concise as possible without being cryptic.

Evolution

I find the best way to start is with the following statement: "I was perfectly fine until…" This should help you focus on the beginning of your current problem. In analyzing the evolution of your condition, take note of how medications may have affected your symptoms. By focusing on the evolution of your medical problems, you begin to organize your observations in a meaningful manner. Sequential, rather than random associations will appear, which may help both you and your physician.

Medications

It's frustrating to have a patient tell a doctor she was given a medication that may have helped or worsened her condition, only she can't remember the name of the drug. "It's a little white pill and it made me sick" simply won't do. Always keep a record of the drugs you take along with their dosage and frequency. If you've forgotten the name of a medication, call the pharmacy or the prescribing doctor's office and ask them to look it up. Are you allergic to any medications? Did this cause changes in your symptoms? If a medication gives you unwanted side effects, make sure your doctor is informed, as different brands of medication may have different profiles when it comes to causing a particular side effect. Be sure to keep a flow chart like the one I have for you in Chapter 7, especially if you are using more than one drug AT THE SAME TIME. Drug combinations can cause serious problems, especially with "specialists" focusing ONLY on their area and failing to inquire about medications and their possible interactions. Always look up your medication on the internet or in the Physicians Desk Reference Book for possible interactions that may explain your complaint.

Be sure to also list ALL over-the-counter medications. Again, these are usually the same as prescription drugs, but at 1/2 the regular dose. This does not mean they have 1/2 the potential side effects or interactions. Don't leave out herbal products. Many contain active ingredients in unregulated strengths, which can inhibit or exaggerate the effectiveness of prescription medication. Finally, list all the vitamin supplements you are currently ingesting. Remove the labels from them and either photocopy or paste them into your medical folder.

Associated Problems

Family diseases and other medical problems interrelate in ways you may never suspect. You should know your family's medical history. Do you have a history of heart disease, elevated cholesterol, high blood pressure, cancer, diabetes, thyroid disease, autoimmune diseases? Do you know the age of your mother when she finished menstruating?

When you were treated for an earlier condition, did the doctor prove the diagnosis or merely surmise the problem? Women tend to be told they have a condition and handed a prescription without the doctor ever doing studies to confirm or deny the diagnosis. That condition may influence your ability to obtain medical health insurance at the best price. Be sure your physician treats you for a real condition whenever possible and not for a probable cause.

Laboratory Work

How many times have you been X-rayed? What did those studies show? If you don't have a copy of the formal (that means typed and signed by the physician) report, you may misinterpret or misrelate the facts to your doctor. Lab tests (again formal printed out copy) are available from hospitals, clinics, or the doctor's office. It is your legal right to have a personal copy of your medical records, including all office notes. You can send a records release request just like the one I have provided in the workbook to these sources. You might be surprised by what you see.

You should list your surgeries and have copies of all operative and pathology reports, along with relevant X ray reports. Some tests need only be done once, which saves you time, money, and often physical discomfort. Be sure to place them in chronological order in your folder so the doctor can easily refer to them during your visit.

Emotion

This is probably the hardest part to learn when visiting a doctor. The plain fact is, most physicians do not deal well with emotional females. They simply want to "look under the hood" and fix the problem. If I were to tell you how differently men and women relate to a doctor, you might not believe me, but here goes: Men speak from fact — women speak first from emotion. A male will come to the office and begin by describing the change in gas mileage in his body, followed by a description of the "sounds" his condition makes. A woman will start with the paint job, the upholstery, and how difficult it was to find a parking space long before she gets to the mileage and sounds. This isn't to say women don't possess all the same information, but we relay it in a different manner. So think like a body mechanic and keep the emotional impact of your condition to the last part of your complaint.

TURNING THE DOCTOR'S HEAD

Doctors make terrible patients and I am no exception. However, I'm going to share with you a personal experience which made me rethink how to negotiate with my doctor to obtain the medical care I felt was right. While writing this workbook, I discovered I had a life-threatening health problem with no obvious complaints, but extraordinary physical findings. After getting over my initial reaction of denial, I focused immediately on the "differential diagnosis" of my condition, and the best test for determining its cause. When I called my doctor regarding the latest laboratory work, I began to "tell" him what I wanted done and discovered he had an immediate negative reaction to it. In the midst of an argument I suddenly realized I had not "asked" for his opinion. As soon as I shifted gears, my doctor was happy to "tell" me his opinion and was now very willing to order a test he would have considered much later in his treatment plan. I had "turned the doctor's head" by giving him time to think his way through the information I had presented. Like a child, he felt it was now HIS idea because I was the one "listening." I had taken the indirect route to power. You can do the same.

Women are natural negotiators, especially when our hormones are in balance. We have higher levels of estrogen, helping us to see things, feel things, and react more clearly in a situation with a personal connection. Male doctors want to focus on immediate solutions to our symptoms and not necessarily the causes. If you doubt me, look at our "prescription addiction." As a patient, you need to redirect your doctor to "see" the tree you've identified in the forest.

HOW TO TELL IF YOUR DOCTOR IS PAYING ATTENTION

I've often heard patients say they just don't think their doctor is listening to them. So how do you tell if your doctor is paying attention to your problem?

I strongly recommend that ALL visits begin in the doctor's office and NOT in an exam room, so that neither of you is naked. It's no mistake that office visits begin under a circumstance that puts you, the patient, in a vulnerable position and on less equal standing. In the office, the doctor is forced to sit, just like you. The idea of having the physician stand in the exam room while the patient asks questions was designed to tell you time is short. How often have you been placed in a room with a drape sheet and had to hail your doctor like a taxi in order to get your questions answered? As a medical student, I was instructed to "keep my hand on the doorknob" to ensure the patient would be "quick" about asking their questions. With the changes in today's health-

care system, this technique has become the hallmark of cost —
contained medicine.

KICKING THE DOCTOR OFF THE CLIFF

When the doctor/patient relationship breaks down, it is
most likely due to "a failure to communicate." So here are eight
warning signs that it's time to kick your doctor off the medical
cliff and find a more caring, interested physician.

You Need to Sharpen Your Heels If:

- Your doctor seldom makes eye contact with you.

- When you offer information that might influence or change
  the diagnosis your doctor has made, he or she rejects it and
  seems to rely solely on his or her expertise.

- The last time you were emotional your doctor maintained a
  polite, unemotional distance.

- When your doctor explains something to you, you get a
  lecture instead of a chance to discuss things you don't
  understand.

- You question your doctor's proposed diagnosis or treatment
  plan, and he or she becomes defensive — or worst of all,
  reminds you who is the doctor.

- After a visit, you felt rushed and failed to mention all of your
  symptoms.

- Your use of a list or other organized method of reporting your observations is not given due consideration, especially if your questions or observations are unusual.
- Your feelings toward your doctor are angry or fearful.

There is no shame in searching for that valuable doctor/patient relationship. Your life could be shorter than you think if you tolerate apathetic care. Remember, physicians are NOT your parents or lovers. They are merely advisors, helping you find YOUR best health. Patients are now extraordinarily educated about the medical process by television, the media, and the internet. Keep looking for that healthy healing relationship. After all, it's only your life.

7

Now it's time to start charting your medical course so you can navigate your way out of hormone hell. I'm going to give you several copies of important forms so you can mark them up as needed.

COLLECTING MEDICAL RECORDS

The first one is a release for a copy of your medical records. Be sure to send one to every physician, hospital, or x-ray facility you have attended. Due to recent confidentiality issues, your insurance carrier no longer provides you with a complete listing of the benefits paid to providers, making it difficult to track down your medical records if you didn't pay your bill with a credit card or by check. Don't forget to contact the medical records department of any hospitals for copies of your inpatient records, laboratory work, operative reports, pathology reports, and any diagnostic studies performed through that facility.

Having trouble obtaining a copy of your own records? Many states have provisions in their Health and Safety Codes that legally allow anyone who can give consent the right to view and obtain copies of their medical records. Here is a sample of the California Health and Safety Code Section 123100:

"Section 123110 of the Health & Safety Code specifically provides that any adult patient, or any minor patient who by law can consent to medical treatment, or any patient representative is entitled to inspect patient records upon written request to a physician and upon payment of reasonable clerical costs to make such records available. The physician must then permit the patient to view his or her records during business hours *within five working days* after receipt of the written request. The patient or patient's representative may be accompanied by one other person of his or her choosing.

The patient or patient's representative is entitled to copies of all or any portion of his or her records that he or she has a right to inspect, upon written request to the physician, along with a fee to defray the cost of copying, not to exceed 25 cents per page or 50 cents per page for records that are copied from microfilm, along with reasonable clerical costs. Physicians must provide patients *with copies within 15 days* of receipt of the request."

As always, it helps to be courteous to office staff, as they are the ones who must facilitate your request. So let's start with a simple medical release form.

Medical Records Release Form

Client Name: _____

Address: _____

City: _____ State: _____ Province: _____

Country: _____ Zip/Postal Code: _____

Telephone: _____ Fax: _____

Email: _____

Date of Birth: _____ Social Security Number: _____

I authorize the release of my medical records or other health care information, including intake forms, chart notes, reports, correspondence, billing statements, and other written information concerning my health and treatment during the period of _____ to _____ ; to be sent to the following person or company.

Client: _____

Address: _____

City: _____ State: _____ Province: _____

Country: _____ Zip/Postal Code: _____

Telephone: _____ Fax: _____

Email: _____

Client Signature: _____ Date: _____

This authorization is valid until: _____date

Now, take your medical scrapbook and start labeling the dividers as follows:

- **Health Concerns** — This section will contain your medical issues along with your observations. Make a new page for each visit, leaving spaces for your handwritten notes during the meeting. Once home, type them up and file in this section.

- **Medical Records** — It's best to do this by specialty, but choose a format that is logical for you to easily locate a record. You may want to subdivide this section into:

  - *X-ray reports* — mammograms, bone density studies

  - *Procedures* — operative reports, colonoscopy reports, EKG studies

  - *Pathology Reports* — don't forget pap smears in this category

  - *Bloodwork* — This area is best managed with a flow sheet. I'll provide you with some examples, but use your spread sheet program to customize one for your particular studies. Remember, different labs use different standards for the same studies, so note the "normal" ranges by your studies.

- *Pharmacy* — Your current medications, how often you take them, and a list of previous medications used to treat various conditions should be listed here. Don't forget to write down ALL over-the-counter products, such as decongestants, vitamins, or stomach soothing products. This works nicely with a spread sheet format.

• **Scientific Articles** — Here is where you keep copies of the relevant research articles your doctor may not have read. Be sure to keep duplicates of any important studies. Abstracts printed from a PubMed search summarizing the findings of an article are sufficient.

Date Drawn					
WBC 4.0-11.0x/uL					
RBC 3.8-5.2x/uL					
Hemoglobin 12-16 g/dL					
Hematocrit 36-48%					
Platelet Count 150-400x/uL					
Neutrophils 45-70%					
Lymphocytes 20-40%					
Monocytes 3-12%					
Eosinophils 0-5%					
Basophils 0-3%					
Sodium 135-147 Eq/L					
Potassium 3.5-5.4 mEq/L					
Chloride 94-110 mEq/L					
CO_2 22-33 mEq/L					
Sed rate <10 Mm/hr					
Triglycerides <200 mg/dl					
Cholesterol, T <200mg/dl					
HDL >34 mg/dl					
LDL 0-130 mg/dl					
Chol/HDLC ratio (coronary risk ratio) Female _ Ave 3.3 Average:4.4 2x Avg : 7.1 3x Avg: 11.0					

Date Drawn					
WBC 4.0-11.0x/uL					
RBC 3.8-5.2x/uL					
Hemoglobin 12-16 g/dL					
Hematocrit 36-48%					
Platelet Count 150-400x/uL					
Neutrophils 45-70%					
Lymphocytes 20-40%					
Monocytes 3-12%					
Eosinophils 0-5%					
Basophils 0-3%					
Sodium 135-147 Eq/L					
Potassium 3.5-5.4 mEq/L					
Chloride 94-110 mEq/L					
CO_2 22-33 mEq/L					
Sed rate <10 Mm/hr					
Triglycerides <200 mg/dl					
Cholesterol, T <200mg/dl					
HDL >34 mg/dl					
LDL 0-130 mg/dl					
Chol/HDLC ratio (coronary risk ratio) Female _ Ave 3.3 Average:4.4 2x Avg : 7.1 3x Avg: 11.0					

Endocrine Lab Reports

Date Drawn	Results	Normal Adult Ranges		
Date of Last Menstrual Cycle				
Day of MC (Day 1 is first day bleeding)				
		Follicular	Luteal	Menopause
STEROIDS				
A'dione ng/ml		0.47-2.68		<1
DHEA ng/ml		5.08-5.51		<5
DHEA-sulfate ug/ml				<0.3
Estradiol pg/ml				5-18
Day 14 Estradiol pg/ml		>200		
Estrone ng/dl		3-10	9-16	
Progesterone Ng/nl		.34-.75	1.0-35	.14-.45
17OH Progesterone ng/ml		0.1-0.8	0.3-3	0.1-0.5
Testosterone ng/ml		0.3-0.9		
Free Testost pg/ml		0.5-3.2	0.5-2.5	0.29-1.73
Pregnenolone ng/dl		10-230		
PROTEINS				
LH IU/ml		1.8-13		0.7-19 11-61
FSH mIU/ml		3-12	2-12	35-151
Prolactin ng/ml		1.9-25.9		1.8-17.9
Insulin uU/ml		5-20 uU/ml uU/mL		
Glucose/insulin ratio mg/uU		<4.5 mg/uU derived		
SHBG Ug/dl		1-3		
THYROID		HYPOTHYROID	EUTHYROID	HYPERTHYROID
TSH ultr uIU/ml		>5.01	0.47-5.01	<0.47
T4 Thyroxine ug/dl		0.7-4.6	4.1-11.1	11.8-46
Free T4 (T7) ng/dl		<0.9	0.9-2.5	>2.5
Free T3 pg/ml		<1.68	1.68-3.54	>3.54
Anti-TG iU/ml		<99		
Anti-TPO iU/ml		<49		
Ferritin ng/ml		12-150		

Endocrine Lab Reports

Date Drawn	Results	Normal Adult Ranges		
Date of Last Menstrual Cycle				
Day of MC (Day 1 is first day bleeding)				
		Follicular	Luteal	Menopause
STEROIDS				
A'dione ng/ml		0.47-2.68	<1	
DHEA ng/ml		5.08-5.51	<5	
DHEA-sulfate ug/ml			<0.3	
Estradiol pg/ml			5-18	
Day 14 Estradiol pg/ml		>200		
Estrone ng/dl		3-10	9-16	
Progesterone Ng/nl		.34-.75	1.0-35	.14-.45
17OH Progesterone ng/ml		0.1-0.8	0.3-3	0.1-0.5
Testosterone ng/ml		0.3-0.9		
Free Testost pg/ml		0.5-3.2	0.5-2.5	0.29-1.73
Pregnenolone ng/dl		10-230		
PROTEINS				
LH IU/ml		1.8-13		0.7-19 11-61
FSH mIU/ml		3-12	2-12	35-151
Prolactin ng/ml		1.9-25.9		1.8-17.9
Insulin uU/ml		5-20 uU/ml uU/mL		
Glucose/insulin ratio mg/uU		<4.5 mg/uU derived		
SHBG Ug/dl		1-3		
THYROID		HYPOTHYROID	EUTHYROID	HYPERTHYROID
TSH ultr uIU/ml		>5.01	0.47-5.01	<0.47
T4 Thyroxine ug/dl		0.7-4.6	4.1-11.1	11.8-46
Free T4 (T7) ng/dl		<0.9	0.9-2.5	>2.5
Free T3 pg/ml		<1.68	1.68-3.54	>3.54
Anti-TG iU/ml		<99		
Anti-TPO iU/ml		<49		
Ferritin ng/ml		12-150		

Medical Records Release Form

Client Name: _____

Address: _____

City: _____ State: _____ Province: _____

Country: _____ Zip/Postal Code: _____

Telephone: _____ Fax: _____

Email: _____

Date of Birth: _____ Social Security Number: _____

I authorize the release of my medical records or other health care information, including intake forms, chart notes, reports, correspondence, billing statements, and other written information concerning my health and treatment during the period of _____ to _____ ; to be sent to the following person or company.

Client: _____

Address: _____

City: _____ State: _____ Province: _____

Country: _____ Zip/Postal Code: _____

Telephone: _____ Fax: _____

Email: _____

Client Signature: _____ Date: _____

This authorization is valid until: _____date

Medical Records Release Form

Client Name: _____

Address: _____

City: _____ State: _____ Province: _____

Country: _____ Zip/Postal Code: _____

Telephone: _____ Fax: _____

Email: _____

Date of Birth: _____ Social Security Number: _____

I authorize the release of my medical records or other health care information, including intake forms, chart notes, reports, correspondence, billing statements, and other written information concerning my health and treatment during the period of _____ to _____ ; to be sent to the following person or company.

Client: _____

Address: _____

City: _____ State: _____ Province: _____

Country: _____ Zip/Postal Code: _____

Telephone: _____ Fax: _____

Email: _____

Client Signature: _____ Date: _____

This authorization is valid until: _____date

		SIALIC ACID POS	FOOD CRAVINGS	INSOMNIA	HEADACHE	FATIGUE	BACKACHE	ACHES/PAINS	CRAMPING	ABD BLOATING	BREAST TENDER	SWOLLEN FEET	SWOLLEN HANDS	CRYING SPELL	ANGER	ANXIETY	DEPRESSION	DAY OF CYCLE
																		1
																		2
																		3
																		4
																		5
																		6
																		7
																		8
																		9
																		10
																		11
																		12
																		13
																		14
																		15
																		16
																		17
																		18
																		19
																		20
																		21
																		22
																		23
																		24
																		25
																		26
																		27
																		28
																		29
																		3
																		3

Medication	Condition treated	Responses/Side Effects

SI Units for Clinical Data (for European Standards)

Conversion:
- to convert from the conventional unit to the SI unit, multiply by the conversion factor;

- to convert from the SI unit to the conventional unit, divide by the conversion factor.

A complete file is available online at
http://jama.ama-assn.org/info/auinst_si.html

Component	Conventional Unit	Conversion Factor	SI Unit
Androstenedione	ng/dL	0.0349	nmol/L
Estradiol	pg/mL	3.671	pmol/L
Estriol	ng/mL	3.467	nmol/L
Estrone	ng/dL	37	pmol/L
Dehydroepiandrosterone (DHEA)	ng/mL	3.47	nmol/L
Progesterone	ng/mL	3.18	nmol/L
Cortisol	µg/dL	27.59	nmol/L
Testosterone	ng/dL	0.0347	nmol/L
Free (T3)	pg/dL	0.0154	pmol/L
Thyrotropin (thyroid-stimulating hormone, TSH)	mIU/L	1.0	mIU/L
Thyroxine, free (T4)	ng/dL	12.87	pmol/L
Ferritin	ng/mL	2.247	pmol/L

Now that your health scrapbook is completely organized, pull up a chair and listen to how other divas have found their way through hormone hell and back. It's all in the next chapter.

8

THE HORMONE DIVA LISTENS

For the past several years, I have been whispering into the ears of thousands of women through my online discussion groups. Although I practiced surgery and women's healthcare for over 15 years and thought I had heard everything, I was not prepared for the hormone horror stories women shared with me from across the nation — and the world. They set my teeth on edge, and gave me a headache from "bonking" my computer screen over and over. However, these stories can teach us ALL the importance of asserting ourselves if we want to be healthy and "sane."

Dear Hormone Diva:

Like others, I have been suffering for many years. I have a great GP but every time I complained about thyroid problems my tests came back "normal." Reading the posts makes me feel good that I am not the only one "suffering."

I demanded my GP refer me to an endocrinologist and what a difference! He calmed my fears of cancer and put me on medication after seeing the lab tests from my GP's office. I am feeling better and better. All I can say is hang in there. Yes — the right doctor is key!

Pal

Dear Hormone Diva:

I used to be a happy, bubbly person and loved to laugh, but all that changed four years ago. I started having strange symptoms: I would be depressed and crying for a few days before my period and my skin would become itchy. I started having very bad neck pain and was told by my first doc that it was stress. Then I developed chest pain, extreme headaches, and my first panic attack. I would wake up at night with such bad panic, not knowing if my kids were in the house or that it was 4AM. The heart palpitations convinced me I was dying.

I found a doc who said I had fibromyalgia and put me on numerous antidepressants, all with no help. So I went to a rheumatologist. Before I entered his office, I had made a list of every symptom, from hair loss, dizziness, headaches, muscle aches, tingling in my hands and feet, memory loss, depression, anxiety, insomnia, heart palps, chest pain, rib pain, burning tongue, fatigue, jaw pain, nausea, and bowel problems. He told me everyone was testing for the wrong things. After a full thyroid panel showed I had Hashimoto's thyroiditis, I was started on meds immediately.

This is what I learned:

- Know your own body, and if something is wrong, don't let some doc tell you it's not. Be persistent and get the answers. Talk to others about how you feel. Someone else has been in the same place and can help you.

- Don't blow off your symptoms — help yourself. There is no such thing as feeling great for years and then going down hill. You need to know why.

- Stay calm. I lost it so many times. Anxiety will make you look like a hypochondriac.

Patty

Dear Hormone Diva:

After two miscarriages at five and six weeks, I gave birth to a healthy boy. Within six weeks, I was so uncomfortable in my own skin I couldn't stand to be with myself. I was having hot flashes and sweating profusely, even when the temperature was in the 40's. My GP did studies and said I had postpartum thyroiditis, but since we were moving to another state, he felt I should follow-up on medication with my new doctors.

I was referred to the endocrinology department by a nurse practitioner, who thought she felt a nodule in the right lobe. They bounced back the referral, stating she could take care of me herself. Over the next eight months, we watched my TSH climb and my FT4 lower and my thyroid become enlarged and painful. I kept gaining weight. However, since the lab values were not "flagged" as abnormal, no treatment was offered.

I became pregnant again and asked for a copy of my "normal labs." I discovered no one had ordered antibodies. I demanded they order them and they came back positive. I was immediately referred back to the endocrinologist, who didn't do anything but doodle when I talked to him. He ignored my abnormal morning cortisol levels and refused to treat me.

I've been through four docs already and fight fatigue on a daily basis. No amount of makeup can hide the tiredness that is evident in my eyes, the windows to my soul.

Rhiannon

Dear Hormone Diva:

I experienced symptoms since puberty of both polycystic ovarian syndrome (insulin resistance) and low thyroid, but my doctors never touched on either. EVER. I was constantly fatigued throughout high school and had to finish my diploma at home. When I was 21 they took some blood and told me my testosterone was a little high, but not to worry. They threw birth control pills at me like candy for the next three years.

Once I stopped the pills to become pregnant, all hell broke loose. I immediately developed a large case of thyroiditis and my insulin resistance started attacking me with a vengenance. I always struggled with facial hair, but now I was growing a beard! I had acne all over and gained 20 pounds. Food felt like poison to me, because every time I ate I had huge reactions — sweating, heart palps, fatigue, ringing in my ears, and headache. I kept drinking coffee to stay awake at work and got into two car accidents during this time.

It took five months to get diagnosed and treated because the endocrinologist just kept taking more tests wanting to "wait and see" if my symptoms would go away. I finally got fed up and went to another doctor who sent me to a reproductive endo specializing in PCOS. I went on supplements and glucophage and have been a real person since.

A good doctor is worth her weight in gold!
Panacea

Dear Hormone Diva:

Reading those medical tests was when I learned to be careful about trusting doctors. I had been told my studies were "fine," "normal." I began to wonder if my internist was interested in my health. I started to argue with her, bringing in articles. She would not read any of them. Finding a doctor willing to prescribe T3 with T4 was not easy. None of the endos in my HMO were willing. One even started shouting that he would not participate in killing his patients! No one was even willing to test my T3 levels.

Due to misdiagnosis, I went a decade without treatment. I went back and got my medical tests from the '90s and found my doctor had only tested my TSH, and it had come back variously at 6 or 7. The top of the range was 5.5. She never told me my studies were abnormal. I think she must have been schooled to believe that any TSH under ten was just "fine," which is the word she kept using. She never tested me for antibodies or T4. I was really shocked to find that she had been so negligent, especially when I was right there telling her about lots of hypo symptoms. I had to get rid of six doctors before I got rid of my symptoms.

Bentley

Dear Hormone Diva:

I ran across one of my old blood tests from 1984 and was astounded to see the TSH range was 0.0-10.0. I was seeing a heart specialist at the time for what I thought were heart symptoms. He couldn't find anything wrong, though I was having palps, PVC's, and one night my heart stopped. My husband couldn't detect a heart beat for several seconds.

It was the complacent attitude of doctors towards my symptoms over the years that led to my seeing a doctor when I became so ill I could barely get out of bed. I had been convinced that my problems were "all in my head" and I should just try harder. I couldn't think. I was phobic about leaving the house. When I finally went for a blood test, my TSH was 119.

Bommer

Dear Hormone Diva:

Yes, I do agree (though it took me 42 years to "see") that the straightest, simplest path to increased health is what you've defined. The toughest part? Breaking free from clinging to old notions, and bad choices that keep one "stuck." But what freedom comes from the disciplines you've outlined. Once I began a "splash" of estradiol, I gained a renewed perspective on just about everything. In essense, I suddenly regained my ability to "get a grip." It's brought about definitive changes in all areas, including personal, and my much stronger focus now allows me to make clearer decisions. Perhaps this is one reason why most male docs just cannot seem to "get it."

Skitterscat

Dear Hormone Diva:

I found a new endo I love. She returns my calls personally and knows me when I come in! We are working together!

Kristine

Dear Hormone Diva:

I often wonder what would have happened if that first Doc back in '96 had done a simple thyroid test. Would I have become as severely hyper as I did? Kicked him off the cliff long ago! Also kicked the first endo over the cliff because he refused to allow any questions and offered no answers...actually got furious at me for asking a simple question. I have a new endo, best money will buy in my area, but the jury is still out on him. He might be on the edge of the cliff, too!

Salem

Dear Hormone Diva:

Three years ago I went to an internist with a major clinic. My complaints were fatigue, depression, constant tinnitus, and I was gaining about four pounds a week even though my eating habits were good. I DEMANDED that he do the thyroid blood test panel. He INSISTED my only problem was depression and prescribed Prozac, which I refused. He ordered my thyroid tests. I had a TSH of 12.71 and very high antibodies. He said my labs looked normal to him and refused to put me on medication.

The next doctor I saw was a family practitioner. My complaints were the same. She put me on thyroid medication and tried to bully me into have a thyroidectomy, even though I didn't have nodules or a goiter. I said I wanted another opinion, so she "fired" me. She had an inefficient staff, calls were never returned, lab specimens lost — it was a nightmare!

I believe every American should have the right to affordable, quality consistent health care. No one should have to lose a good doctor because of their health insurance or put up with shoddy care.

CurlyWings

Dear Hormone Diva:

About four years ago my doctor tested my TSH because I was gaining weight. He said it was fine and that my lethargy and weight gain was due to "getting older and not taking time to eat right or exercise." I got angry with myself. Why was I insisting on blaming a gland, when it was obvious to the doctor that it was my own lack of desire to stay healthy which was to blame? I got a second opinion and was told the weight was due to a lack of caring on my part, and my age. Two doctors, one opinion — it was ME. I was a failure. It was very lonely and degrading.

I found a local endocrinologist who understood and did the right tests. We're working to get my thyroid to a place where we can coexist peacefully. Those other doctors were right on one count. Our health IS our responsibility, which is why so many of us have taken our last ounce of self-esteem, energy and HOPE to fight our way to where we are now — on the road to recovery. The most horrible part of this nightmare was not being BELIEVED, not being given credit for knowing my own body, and just being passed off as "just another aging female who doesn't want to take charge of her health."
Kymba

Dear Hormone Diva:

I developed pneumonia, but never seemed to recover. I had terrible fatigue, dry skin, weight gain, and I mentioned I hadn't had a period in two years. This is where things get really scary and ugly. The internal medicine doctor comes in, listens to me and then begins to argue with me over my family history that is recorded in my chart. I finally told him to accept the fact it was inaccurate. He was consumed with the fact I did not have a period and I had to keep redirecting him back to my primary complaint — fatigue. He says my blood work is normal. Then he literally whips out his palm pilot and begins to plug in my complaints and tells me his palm pilot tells him that I suffer from depression and sleep apnea. Another doctor reviews the lab work and says there are abnormalities there and sends me back to this doctor. When I ask why HE said they were normal, he responded "nothing was flagged" on the report and everything is within acceptable range. My TSH was at 4.4, but he claims I don't have a problem because it is not at 5. He recommends I purchase a can of bag balm for my dry skin. He also decides, based upon his palm pilot, that I suffer from PCOS and decides I should see an OB/GYN.

I came home and spent the weekend reading everything I could find on the internet about thyroid disease. I spent the following Monday calling every endo in town until I found one who would see me without a referral. As I spoke with the doctor I realized he was actually listening to me and was not intimidated by my knowledge of the problem. I am so glad I took matters into my own hands.

Mako

Dear Hormone Diva:

Although I have a Ph.D from an Ivy League University, my brain was working poorly. I started having to look at a phone number three or four times while dialing, and still made mistakes. I cried when we suddenly had to dial the area code in addition to the seven digit number for local numbers! Here is what I learned: Healing takes a long time.

Getting well requires a partnership with your doctor and other health care practitioners, and not all docs have the same standards or training.

Annette

Dear Hormone Diva:

Nothing is easy. You have to be in charge of your health, knowledgeable about your options, and able to stand up to doctors. I have changed doctors three times over the years. Women need to manage their own journey through these stressful hormonal times. Not feeling helpless and being in charge is half the battle.

VSW6

Dear Hormone Diva:

The forgotten side to the overall detrimental effects of autoimmune disease has to do with the emotional toll it quietly takes on incapacitated victims. Part of the price we pay for the typically invisible pain and suffering we experience extends not only to pleading with our doctors for understanding, but wearily trying to communicate our needs to spouses, children and family members. Fighting against feeling worn-out with fatigue, we sense we're aging faster than we should. It's an unrelenting battle fought everyday because we don't know what to expect, what can be accomplished, or how much tolerance we ourselves can extend. We're fed up with the devastation of antibodies wreaking havoc with our bodies, our emotions, and even our relationships. The dimming of our energy robs the lightness from our lives and makes our days a struggle, rather than an adventure. So much is lost when the chance to be your best is replaced by feeling like you're 80 years old...

I wanted to share with you a way I found I was able to get around a doctor's "No." My last appointment wasn't with the top doc endo, but with his nurse practitioner. I went carrying with me the results of some blood lab tests pertinent to what I wanted her to focus on in the appointment. These had been previously ordered by the naturopath and my gynecologist. While handing tests to her measuring estrogen, TSH, etc., I was able to present a brief summation of my current symptoms and request what new studies I'd like done in conjunction with what she was looking at and why. She didn't balk, nor did she appear to feel overwhelmed as some often do when there is a lot of ground to cover — mostly, I think because my words were being bolstered by the "legitimacy" of tests being performed by another professional in a related field. She didn't have to think twice, handed me four separate sheets for new lab work to be done over a three month period — and all with a smile. WOW!

Stef

Dear Hormone Diva:

I fully resent these "dinosaur" doctors that can't see two feet beyond their nose when it comes to treating women with respect. They assume because we are women, we are hysterical and know-nothings. When I asked my doctor what he was doing if not prescribing estrogen, he said "lots and lots of soy and anti-depressants." He'd be off that cliff in a heartbeat, if I didn't need him for mundane things like bronchitis, etc.

I so wish I could find someone who would agree to the tests and prescriptions that I want. I'm not stupid. I've done a major amount of research and I DO know more than my doctor regarding thyroid and menopause. He has the sheepskin hanging on his wall, so he has license to tell me what I need and don't need. I want to be in charge of my own health. Period. End of sentence! It's a cold, cruel world out there regarding this so called medical profession and a sad state of affairs that we have to beg and plead for ways to help ourselves regain the health we have a God given right to. Off the soapbox now.

Gayle

As you can see, it's important to keep looking for that important partnership with your healthcare provider. In a recent advice column, "Tell Me About It," by Carolyn Hax, she wrote: "I think anyone who doesn't assert himself is going to get inadequate care, regardless of how good the doctor is. If the doctor says it's in your head, ask for another opinion. If the doc says meds, ask about counseling. If the doc says counseling, ask about meds. Ask to see a specialist. Ask ask ask. And if you feel rushed or intimidated by your doctor, get another doctor."

But what if you're unable to find that "perfect match?" What if you can't get past "NO!" Frustration leads to invention and ingenuity, so follow me to the next chapter and discover The Hormone Diva Survival Kit.

9

THE HORMONE DIVA SURVIVAL KIT

I tend to let my imagination wander when faced with impossible situations and picture myself alone on an island with nothing more than my cell phone, laptop or PDA and a mail/package delivery system. After all, this IS a civilized island — I created it! How would I keep myself healthy until a cruise ship steams by and rescues me? Not to worry. I'll create The Hormone Diva Survival Kit.

First, I would take out my Health Scrapbook and make sure all the information was complete and accurate. Next, I would get on the internet and order the following items:

1) An automatic digital Blood Pressure unit. Hypertension is a silent killer, and if you don't monitor your blood pressure during hormone changes, you could be damaging your kidneys, heart or lungs. I prefer the wrist units for size, ease of use, and storage of data. Go online and search for "digital wrist BP" and compare prices for the various units.

2) The Donna Salivary Ovulation Tester. This little unit is the size of a lipstick and can predict if you're ovulating or not. You'll need this to time mid-cycle estradiol levels or to confirm you ovulated for each cycle. Numerous outlets sell this product.

3) Digital basal thermometer. Basal body temps can help determine if you are hypothyroid, in addition to serving as a secondary source for predicting ovulation.

4) Biosafe screening kits for TSH, cholesterol, Hemoglobin A1c. Just a little prick of blood and you can obtain a wealth of information. These tests are available online at a discount by ordering from

http://www. menopausediet.com/Store/biosafe.htm

5) Stool guiac tests. These are the same test kits used by doctors to detect blood in the stool, an early sign of colon cancer. They are produced by several companies.

6) Urine dipsticks for glucose and ketones. Ketoacidosis can rob your bones of calcium, and should be avoided if you want to stay a healthy Diva. Any leakage of glucose in the urine should be confirmed by a blood test. There are several blood glucose monitoring systems available.

7) No Hormone Diva Survival Kit would be complete without a copy of either The Menopause Diet or The Goddess Diet Book.

Now I would save in my Favorites file of my browser the following links:

The National Library of Medicine (PubMed)

http://www4.ncbi.nlm.nih.gov/entrez/query.fcgi

PubMed, a service of the National Library of Medicine, provides access to over 12 million MEDLINE citations back to the mid-1960's and additional life science journals. The best way to search is to put in your topic+second topic, such as thyroid+ferritin. You can read the abstract of any article and determine if you want a full reprint. If so, sign up for Lonesome Doc.

http://www.nlm.nih.gov/loansomedoc/loansome_home.html

Loansome Doc allows users to order full-text copies of articles from a medical library delivered either online or to your door. You must register to use this service, and most articles cost approximately $10 per copy. Full instructions are on the site.

Medline Plus

http://www.nlm.nih.gov/medlineplus/

This site lists clinical trial information and offers a long list of resources for the public.

WebMD

http://my.webmd.com/medical_information/drug_and_herb/default.htm

An excellent resource. I like the drug and herb database for looking up possible interactions.

HealthCheckUSA

http://menopausediet.com/Store/healthcheck.htm

You can order the same tests physicians prescribe, and they are performed by an accredited laboratory. You can do a search for "internet blood screening laboratories" to find other companies.

The Menopause Diet

http://www.menopausediet.com

Companion site to The Hormone Diva (http://www.hormonediva.com) and an excellent source for information about menopause and how hormones affect our ability to lose weight.

Masters Marketing

http://www.mastersmarketing.com

An excellent source for medications manufactured overseas by the same US companies. One of the few sources for the French 17β estradiol product, Oestrogel. Please read the FDA FAQ on buying medicines and medical products online.

http://www.fda.gov/oc/buyonline/faqs.html

Cleveland Clinic Eclinic

http://www.clevelandclinic.org/services/eclinic.htm

e-Cleveland Clinic is a web-based extension of the clinic's role as a respected referral institution. It is one of the few sites offering second opinions without the need for a physician referral. You can do a search in your browser using "online medical second opinions" to find other institutions.

TRIAGE

Now, using my copy of this workbook, I would write out my symptoms, and check them against the list of related symptoms for thyroid, adrenal, or ovarian problems. After deciding which system might be out of balance, I would reach into my survival kit, or call up the online laboratory and order the recommended screening tests for this condition. In the meantime, I would review my food and exercise profile, and decide if adding another lap around the coconut palm each day in addition to my usual stress reduction therapy would be of benefit. Of course, I would have my well-underlined copy of The Menopause Diet or The Goddess Diet book in my bag. Once I received my test results, I would compile the information and do an online search through PubMed for the latest recommended therapies. If I felt comfortable with the information, I might proceed to ordering a small amount of the medication for this condition. I would keep a log of my observations and repeat any studies to determine if my values were changing in the right direction. Finally, I could assemble all my data and order an online consultation from one of the departments at a major university.

THE HORMONE DIVA SPEAKS

Sometimes you just need a little "food for thought" from a friend. That's where the Hormone Diva, your personal health coach, can help. No need to feel rushed, embarrassed or made to wait when help is just an email away. So pull up a chair, have a cup of tea (with a shot of sympathy on the side), and hear my words of Diva wisdom.

Dear Hormone Diva:

My doctor started me on the patch for my hormones, but I'm still having hot flashes. What's wrong?

MJ

It may be you're not able to absorb the estradiol in the patch. First, don't use a patch if you are an avid hot tubber, as the hot water can cause the patch to "dump" its contents all at once. If you take medication, such as SSRI's (Celexa, Effexor), these can affect the sympathetic tone in your skin, making it difficult to vasodilate enough to pick up the medication. If you want to know the answer, put on a patch, and get a blood estradiol level done about four hours later. It should be around 70-114 pg/ml. If not, you are not able to "get" the medication from the patch. Ask to switch to either the estrogel (Oestrogel) from Europe or an oral form. Again, always check with a blood estradiol level to be sure you are absorbing and breaking down the medication properly.

Dear Hormone Diva:

I've heard estrogen affects my thyroid medication. Can you explain?

Trisha

Estradiol affects thyroid binding globulin, making less of your medication "free" to work in your tissue. Many women need to adjust their thyroid medication once they get their estradiol levels in range. So, make sure your estradiol is between 70-114 pg/ml, and then recheck your thyroid studies, such as TSH. You may need a 25% increase in your thyroid medication.

Dear Hormone Diva:

My doctor scared me and said he wouldn't give me estrogen unless I took progesterone daily. Otherwise I would get uterine cancer. Is this true?

Melanie

Your doctor is referring to studies done with synthetic estrogens that were not monitored by blood levels. Recent studies with estradiol have shown low dose levels (defined as a blood estradiol level between 70-114 pg/ml) do not stimulate the uterine lining. However, the use of vaginal progesterone for five days every four months will cause you to shed the lining of the uterus if any developed. This prevents endometrial hyperplasia, the pre-cancerous changes in the lining. Taking progesterone or progestins daily can cause weight gain, insulin resistance, and a whole lot of other problems.

Dear Hormone Diva:

My doctor is dead set against my taking estrogen alone, so he gave me a prescription that contains estrogen and progesterone combined. What can I do?

Gina

First, you were given a prescription for synthetic estrogen and progestins, NOT natural estrogen and progesterone. You already know this combo was found to increase the risk of breast cancer, and didn't offer any protection for your heart, brain or bones. So, here is what I suggest you do. Ask your doctor for two prescriptions: estradiol, and the progestin. Make them separate prescriptions. Then, fill just the estradiol. I know…but there are no pharmacy police. Just be sure your estradiol level is low (no more than .5mg), and then fill the progestin and use it only for five days with the estradiol. Keep using the estradiol until you have a period, which should be in two days. Then stop BOTH medications until you stop bleeding. Restart the estradiol only again for the next few months and repeat.

Dear Hormone Diva:

I've heard that estrogen and thyroid meds shouldn't be taken together. What is the best time to take them?

Myna

Ideally, you want to separate the drugs by about four to six hours. Some women find it easier to take their thyroid meds in the morning and their estradiol at night. See what works for you.

Dear Hormone Diva:

My doctor wants me to use DHEA and pregnenolone to boost my energy. I've heard this might cause me problems. What do you think?

Treena

Well, I think your doctor is into the "anti-aging" concept of meds. DHEA in women orally can lower our HDL, the good cholesterol levels. It raises testosterone, but doesn't do much for estradiol. Pregnenolone increases androgens, or male hormones in our bodies. So, using them to fight "fatigue" is like taking steroids. You FEEL better, but you are creating new problems. Now, if you had your ovaries removed and show NO testosterone, DHEA as a transdermal cream would be a good idea. Ask your doctor to prescribe the cream form. Usual dose is 25mg a day.

Dear Hormone Diva:

Instead of a regular period, I get some brown spotting and only for a couple of days. Should I get an FSH done to see if I am in menopause?

Marsha

Actually, brown spotting says you didn't ovulate that month, which may or may not indicate menopause, etc. The answer lies in first checking with the salivary sialic acid tester (The Donna) to see if you "fern." If you fail to "fern" repeatedly, then get an FSH done on the days you spot. If the FSH is above 20, you are in perimenopause and should consider low dose estradiol therapy. Realize, the later you start estradiol therapy, the more sensitivity is lost in the cells. We need them to respond to estradiol in order to keep our blood vessels elastic, our eyes clear of cataracts and our bones strong.

Dear Hormone Diva:

My doctor has given me Triest but he won't test my blood estradiol levels. I don't like using something I can't monitor.
Denise

I think you are very smart. First, Triest is a cream and that means practically NOTHING of estradiol gets transported across your skin. Estradiol has to be in a gel in order to penetrate the skin. I'm not surprised he won't test your blood, because it would show NO CHANGE. You can order your own estradiol levels before and after using the Triest and see what you find. Go back to him with the results and see if this changes his mind. If not, kick him off the medical cliff and get another doctor!

Dear Hormone Diva:

My family doctor diagnosed me with "clinical depression", even though my thyroid studies showed I had Hashis. After three docs, I got put on Synthroid, but I feel like I am crawling out of my skin! I've been through four docs, and they all seem to believe that a Synthroid a day should make me feel fine. I know my body, and this has been a run-around for years. It's not in my head. It's on their lab sheets.

Destiny

Sweetie...You're a walking low ferritin, low adrenal, hypothyroid poster child, also known as polyglandular syndrome type 2, so sharpen your heels, kick those arrogant docs off the medical cliff, and DEMAND 21 hydroxylase antibodies, ACA, serum ferritin, as your hyper anxiety response to thyroid meds is due to low serum ferritin compounded by the adrenal issues.

CAN WE TALK?

Absolutely. As you can see, women just need a bit of direction and support when it comes to taking charge of their own health. So if you feel you want to talk with someone who understands what you're going through, visit my website http://www.hormonediva.com.

You'll find articles on the latest "hot" medical topics, health reports, including my free newsletter Larrian Reports, links to my other sites on nutrition (Menopausediet.com, Goddessdiet.com, Gladiatordiet.com) and a discussion board for members only. If you're in need of a little one-on-one with a personal health coach, The Hormone Diva will help you design your hormone recovery program with innovative ways for getting the most for your health dollar. Think of it as a guilt-free, no nagging plan designed to bring out the hidden diva in you!

FOLLOW YOUR INTUTITION

I hope this workbook has given you the courage to follow your own intuition when it comes to your body. After all, it's more accurate than a five-minute office visit with an overworked doctor. As women, we constantly seek approval from others. But when it comes to your health, only you can pass judgement on how well you've done. It just takes the courage to say "no" to indifferent care.

So, the next time you feel stuck in "hormone hell," just remember: You're Not Crazy...It's Your Hormones!

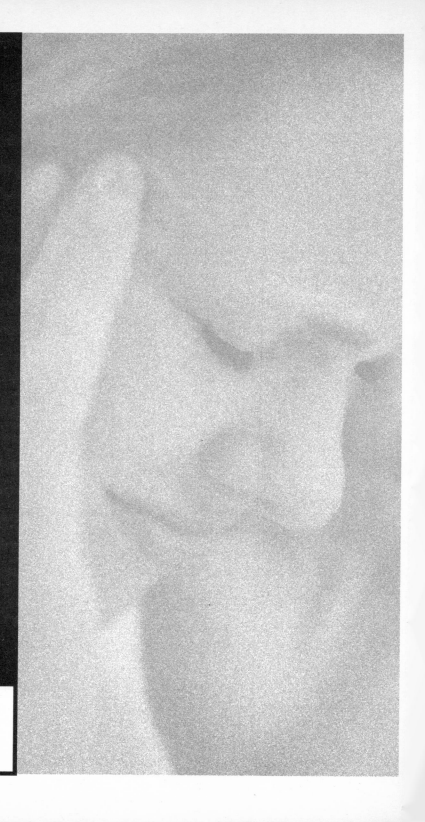

BIBLIOGRAPHY

1.	Presser, H., *Temporal data relating to the menstrual cycle, in Biorhythms and Human Reproduction,* H.F. Ferin M, Richart RM et al eds, Editor. 1974, John Wiley and Sons: New York. p. 145-160.

2.	Oster, G. and S.L. Yang, *Cyclic variation of sialic acid content in saliva.* Am J Obstet Gynecol, 1972. 114(2): p. 190-3.

3.	Guida, M., *et al., Salivary ferning and the menstrual cycle in women.* Clin Exp Obstet Gynecol, 1993. 20(1): p. 48-54.

4.	Calamera, J.C., O. Vilar, and R. Nicholson, *Changes in sialic acid concentration in human saliva during the menstrual cycle.* Int J Fertil, 1986. 31(1): p. 43-5.

5.	Hollowell, J.G., *et al., Serum TSH, T(4), and thyroid antibodies in the United States population (1988 to 1994): National Health and Nutrition Examination Survey (NHANES III).* J Clin Endocrinol Metab, 2002. 87(2): p. 489-99.

6.	De Groot, L., *Dangerous dogmas in medicine: the nonthyroidal illness syndrome.* Journal of Clinical Endocrinology and Metabolism, 1999. 84(1): p. 151-164.

7.	Bunevicius, R., *et al., Effects of thyroxine as compared with thyroxine plus triiodothyronine in patients with hypothyroidism.* N Engl J Med, 1999. 340(6): p. 424-9.

8.	Knight., L., *et al., Delayed gastric emptying and decreased antral contractility in normal premenopausal women compared with men.* Am J Gastroenterol, 1997. 92(6): p. 968-75.

9.	Maes, M., *et al., Components of biological variation, including seasonality, in blood concentrations of TSH, TT3, FT4, PRL, cortisol and testosterone in healthy volunteers.* Clin Endocrinol (Oxf), 1997. 46(5): p. 587-98.

10.	Arafah, B.M., *Increased need for thyroxine in women with hypothyroidism during estrogen therapy.* N Engl J Med, 2001. 344(23): p. 1743-9.

11.	Gartner, R., *et al., Selenium supplementation in patients with autoimmune thyroiditis decreases thyroid peroxidase antibodies concentrations.* J Clin Endocrinol Metab, 2002. 87(4): p. 1687-91.

12.	Hess, S.Y., *et al., Iron deficiency anemia reduces thyroid peroxidase activity in rats.* J Nutr, 2002. 132(7): p. 1951-5.

13.	Facchini, F.S., *Effect of phlebotomy on plasma glucose and insulin concentrations.* Diabetes Care, 1998. 21(12): p. 2190.

14.	Shakir, K.M., *et al., Anemia: a cause of intolerance to thyroxine sodium.* Mayo Clin Proc, 2000. 75(2): p. 189-92.

15.   Ditta, A., *et al., Significance of thyrotrophin and thyroxine estimations in type 1 diabetes.* J Pak Med Assoc, 2001. 51(10): p. 349-51.

16.   Divi, R.L., H.C. Chang, and D.R. Doerge, *Anti-thyroid isoflavones from soybean: isolation, characterization, and mechanisms of action.* Biochem Pharmacol, 1997. 54(10): p. 1087-96.

17.   Cassidy, A., S. Bingham, and K.D. Setchell, *Biological effects of a diet of soy protein rich in isoflavones on the menstrual cycle of premenopausal women.* Am J Clin Nutr, 1994. 60(3): p. 333-40.

18.   Patisaul, H.B., *et al., Soy isoflavone supplements antagonize reproductive behavior and estrogen receptor alpha- and beta-dependent gene expression in the brain.* Endocrinology, 2001. 142(7): p. 2946-52.

19.   Konno, N., *et al., Association between dietary iodine intake and prevalence of subclinical hypothyroidism in the coastal regions of Japan.* J Clin Endocrinol Metab, 1994. 78(2): p. 393-7.

20.   Reinhardt, W., *et al., Effect of small doses of iodine on thyroid function in patients with Hashimoto's thyroiditis residing in an area of mild iodine deficiency [see comments].* Eur J Endocrinol, 1998. 139(1): p. 23-8.

21.   Zhu, X.Y., *et al., Endemic goiter due to iodine rich salt and its pickled vegetables.* Chin Med J (Engl), 1984. 97(7): p. 545-8.22. Farrar, G.E., Jr., *Goiter, iodine, and cabbage.* Clin Ther, 1990. 12(2): p. 191-2.

23.   McLaren, E.H. and W.D. Alexander, *Goitrogens.* Clin Endocrinol Metab, 1979. 8(1): p. 129-44.

24.   Kosovskii, M.I., *et al., [Glucose tolerance disorders in patients with hypothyroidism].* Probl Endokrinol (Mosk), 1992. 38(2): p. 26-9.

25.   Kelly, G.S., *Peripheral metabolism of thyroid hormones: a review.* Altern Med Rev, 2000. 5(4): p. 306-33.

26.   De Lorenzo, F., *et al., Chronic fatigue syndrome: physical and cardiovascular deconditioning.* Qjm, 1998. 91(7): p. 475-81.

27.   Chen, A.Y., *et al., The development of breast carcinoma in women with thyroid carcinoma.* Cancer, 2001. 92(2): p. 225-31.

28.   Mettler FA, J., Guiberteau MJ, *Techniques for Imaging theThyroid, in Essentials of Nuclear Medicine Imaging.* 1998, W. B. Saunders: Philadelphia. p. 112-116.

29.   Williams, G.H. and R.G. Dluhy, *Diseases of the Adrenal Gland, in Harrison's Principles of Internal Medicine.* 1994, McGraw-Hill Inc: Philadelphia.

30.   Bakalov, V.K., *et al., Adrenal antibodies detect asymptomatic auto-immune adrenal insufficiency in young women with spontaneous premature*

ovarian failure. Hum Reprod, 2002. 17(8): p. 2096-100.

31. Kasperlik-Zaluska, A.A., *et al., Secondary adrenal insufficiency associated with autoimmune disorders: a report of twenty-five cases.* Clin Endocrinol (Oxf), 1998. 49(6): p. 779-83.

32. Degros, V., *et al., [21-hydroxylase autoantibodies as a marker of adrenal involvement in patients with autoimmune endocrinopathies].* Ann Biol Clin (Paris), 1999. 57(6): p. 705-9.

33. Chen, S., *et al., Autoantibodies to steroidogenic enzymes in autoimmune polyglandular syndrome, Addison's disease, and premature ovarian failure.* J Clin Endocrinol Metab, 1996. 81(5): p. 1871-6.

34. Valentino, R., *et al., Unusual association of thyroiditis, Addison's disease, ovarian failure and celiac disease in a young woman.* J Endocrinol Invest, 1999. 22(5): p. 390-4.

35. Niepomniszcze, H., *et al., Primary thyroid disorders in endogenous Cushing's syndrome.* Eur J Endocrinol, 2002. 147(3): p. 305-11.

36. Papanicolaou, D.A., *et al., Nighttime Salivary Cortisol: A Useful Test for the Diagnosis of Cushing's Syndrome.* J Clin Endocrinol Metab, 2002. 87(10): p. 4515-21.

37. Nakajima, S.T. and M. Gibson, *The effect of a meal on circulating steady-state progesterone levels.* J Clin Endocrinol Metab, 1989. 69(4): p. 917-9.

38. Shirtcliff, E.A., *et al., Use of salivary biomarkers in biobehavioral research: cotton-based sample collection methods can interfere with salivary immunoassay results.* Psychoneuroendocrinology, 2001. 26(2): p. 165-73.

39. Girdler, S.S., C.A. Pedersen, and K.C. Light, *Thyroid axis function during the menstrual cycle in women with premenstrual syndrome.* Psychoneuroendocrinology, 1995. 20(4): p. 395-403.

40. Caron, P., *et al., Effects of hyperthyroidism on binding proteins for steroid hormones.* Clin Endocrinol (Oxf), 1989. 31(2): p. 219-24.

41. Glinoer, D., *et al., Effects of estrogen on thyroxine-binding globulin metabolism in rhesus monkeys.* Endocrinology, 1977. 100(1): p. 9-17.

42. Sayegh, R., *et al., The effect of a carbohydrate-rich beverage on mood, appetite, and cognitive function in women with premenstrual syndrome.* Obstet Gynecol, 1995. 86(4 Pt 1): p. 520-8.

43. Hansen, C.M., J.E. Leklem, and L.T. Miller, *Vitamin B-6 status indicators decrease in women consuming a diet high in pyridoxine glucoside.* J Nutr, 1996. 126(10): p. 2512-8.

44. Marx, T. and A. Mehta, *Polycystic Ovary Syndrome: Pathogenesis and treatment over the short and long term.* Cleveland Clinic Journal of Medicine, 2003. 70(1): p. 31-45.

45.   Gonzalez, F., *Adrenal involvement in polycystic ovary syndrome.* Semin Reprod Endocrinol, 1997. 15(2): p. 137-57.

46.   Goudas, V.T. and D.A. Dumesic, *Polycystic ovary syndrome.* Endocrinol Metab Clin North Am, 1997. 26(4): p. 893-912.

47.   Timpatanapong, P. and A. Rojanasakul, *Hormonal profiles and prevalence of polycystic ovary syndrome in women with acne.* J Dermatol, 1997. 24(4): p. 223-9.

48.   Dixon, J.B. and P.E. O'Brien, *Neck circumference a good predictor of raised insulin and free androgen index in obese premenopausal women: changes with weight loss.* Clin Endocrinol (Oxf), 2002. 57(6): p. 769-78.

49.   Rebora, A., *Telogen effluvium: an etiopathogenetic theory.* Int J Dermatol., 1993. 32(5): p. 339-40.

50.   Shum, K., D. Cullum, and A. Messenger, *Hair loss in women with hyperandrogenism: Four cases responding to finasteride.* J AAD, 2002. 47(5): p. 733-9.

51.   Barth, J.H., et al., *Spironolactone is an effective and well tolerated systemic antiandrogen therapy for Hirsute women.* J Clin Endocrinol Metab, 1989. 68(5): p. 966-70.

52.   Polson, D.W., H.D. Mason, and S. Franks, *Bromocriptine treatment of women with clomiphene-resistant polycystic ovary syndrome.* Clin Endocrinol (Oxf), 1987. 26(2): p. 197-203.

53.   Steinberger, E., et al., *Glucocorticoid therapy in hyperandrogenism.* Baillieres Clin Obstet Gynaecol, 1990. 4(3): p. 457-71.

54.   Gleicher, N., et al., *Is endometriosis an autoimmune disease?* Obstet Gynecol, 1987. 70(1): p. 115-22.

55.   Grosskinsky, C.M. and J. Halme, *Endometriosis: the host response.* Baillieres Clin Obstet Gynaecol, 1993. 7(4): p. 701-13.

56.   DePriest, P.D., et al., *Transvaginal sonography as a screening method for the detection of early ovarian cancer.* Gynecol Oncol, 1997. 65(3): p. 408-14.

57.   Cummings, A.M. and J.L. Metcalf, *Effects of estrogen, progesterone, and methoxychlor on surgically induced endometriosis in rats.* Fundam Appl Toxicol, 1995. 27(2): p. 287-90.

58.   Kester, M.H., et al., *Potent inhibition of estrogen sulfotransferase by hydroxylated metabolites of polyhalogenated aromatic hydrocarbons reveals alternative mechanism for estrogenic activity of endocrine disrupters.* J Clin Endocrinol Metab, 2002. 87(3): p. 1142-50.

59.   Michnovicz, J., *Environmental modulation of oestrogen metabolism in humans.* Int Clin Nutr Rev, 1987. 7: p. 169-173.

60.   Takeda, R., *et al., Schmidt's syndrome: autoimmune polyglandular disease of the adrenal and thyroid glands.* Isr Med Assoc J, 1999. 1(4): p. 285-6.

61.   Leedman, P.J., et al., *Thyroid hormone modulates the interaction between iron regulatory proteins and the ferritin mRNA iron-responsive element.* J Biol Chem, 1996. 271(20): p. 12017-23.

62.   Takamatsu, J., *et al., Serum ferritin as a marker of thyroid hormone action on peripheral tissues.* J Clin Endocrinol Metab, 1985. 61(4): p. 672-6.

63.   *Risks and benefits of estrogen plus progestin in healthy postmenopausal women: principal results From the Women's Health Initiative randomized controlled trial.* Jama, 2002. 288(3): p. 321-33.

64.   DeLignieres, B., *Hormone replacement therapy compliance and individually adapted doses.* 7th International Congress on Menopause, ed. B. Von Schoultz and C. Christiansen. 1993, Stockholm: Casterton, Parthenon Publishing Group. 59-67.

65.   Weaver, C.M., *et al., Impact of exercise on bone health and contraindication of oral contraceptive use in young women.* Med Sci Sports Exerc, 2001. 33(6): p. 873-80.

66.   Shirtcliff, E.A., *et al., Assessing estradiol in biobehavioral studies using saliva and blood spots: simple radioimmunoassay protocols, reliability, and comparative validity.* Horm Behav, 2000. 38(2): p. 137-47.

67.   Fishman, J., J. Schneider, and R.e.a. Hershcopf, *Increased estrogen 16alpha-hydroxylase activity in women with breast and endometrial cancer.* J Steroid Biochem, 1984. 20: p. 1077-1081.

68.   Bucala, R., *et al., Increased levels of 16 alpha-hydroxyestrone-modified proteins in pregnancy and in systemic lupus erythematosus.* J Clin Endocrinol Metab, 1985. 60(5): p. 841-7.

69.   Whitehead, M.I., *Prevention of endometrial abnormalities.* Acta Obstet Gynecol Scand Suppl, 1986. 134: p. 81-91.

70.   Weiderpass, E., *et al., Low-potency oestrogen and risk of endometrial cancer: a case-control study.* Lancet, 1999. 353(9167): p. 1824-8.

71.   Morreal, C.E., *et al., Urinary excretion of estrone, estradiol, and estriol in postmenopausal women with primary breast cancer.* J Natl Cancer Inst, 1979. 63(5): p. 1171-4.

72.   Jones, K.P., *Estrogens and progestins: what to use and how to use it.* Clin Obstet Gynecol, 1992. 35(4): p. 871-83.

73.   Taylor, M., *Alternatives to conventional hormone replacement therapy.* Compr Ther, 1997. 23(8): p. 514-32.

74.   Simon, J.A., *et al., The absorption of oral micronized progesterone: the effect of food, dose proportionality, and comparison with intramuscular progesterone.* Fertil Steril, 1993. 60(1): p. 26-33.

75.   Nahoul, K., *et al., Profiles of plasma estrogens, progesterone and their metabolites after oral or vaginal administration of estradiol or progesterone.* Maturitas, 1993. 16(3): p. 185-202.

76.   Bourgain, C., *et al., Effects of natural progesterone on the morphology of the endometrium in patients with primary ovarian failure.* Hum Reprod, 1990. 5(5): p. 537-43.

77.   Kim, S., *et al., Antiproliferative effects of low-dose micronized progesterone.* Fertil Steril, 1996. 65(2): p. 323-31.

78.   Miles, R.A., *et al., Pharmacokinetics and endometrial tissue levels of progesterone after administration by intramuscular and vaginal routes: a comparative study.* Fertil Steril, 1994. 62(3): p. 485-90.

79.   Lee, J.R., *Osteoporosis reversal with transdermal progesterone.* Lancet, 1990. 336(8726): p. 1327.

80.   Leonetti, H.B., S. Longo, and J.N. Anasti, *Transdermal progesterone cream for vasomotor symptoms and postmenopausal bone loss.* Obstet Gynecol, 1999. 94(2): p. 225-8.

81.   Lee, J., *What Your Doctor May Not Tell You About Menopause: The Breakthrough Book on Natural Progesterone.* 1996: Warner Books.

82.   Lee, J., *Natural Progesterone: The Multiple Roles of a remarkable Hormone.* 1993, Sebastopol: BLL Publishing.

83.   Haines, C.J., *et al., The perception of the menopause and the climacteric among women in Hong Kong and southern China.* Prev Med, 1995. 24(3): p. 245-8.

84.   Murkies, A., *Phytoestrogens - what is the current knowledge?* Aust. Fam Physician, 1998. 27(suppl 1): p. 547-551.

85.   Notelovitz, M., *Individualizing Hormone Therapy: Principles and Practice,* 2001, Medscape.

86.   Ettinger, B., A. Pressman, and A. Van Gessel, *Low-dosage esterified estrogens opposed by progestin at 6-month intervals.* Obstet Gynecol, 1991. 98(2): p. 205-211.

87.   Lobo, R., *et al., Effects of lower doses of conjugated equine estrogens and medroxyprogesterone acetate on plasma lipids and lipoproteins, coagulation factors, and carbohydrate metabolism.* Fertil Steril, 2001. 76(1): p. 13-24.

88. Smith-Bindman, R., *et al.*, *Endovaginal ultrasound to exclude endometrial cancer and other endometrial abnormalities.* Jama, 1998. 280(17): p. 1510-7.

89. Murphy, A.A., *et al.*, *Regression of uterine leiomyomata in response to the antiprogesterone RU 486.* J Clin Endocrinol Metab, 1993. 76(2): p. 513-7.

90. Turner, R. and e. al, *Is Resveratrol an Estrogen Agonist in Growing Rats?* Endocrinology, 1999. 140: p. 50-54.

91. Luborsky, J., *et al.*, *Ovarian antibodies, FSH and inhibin B: independent markers associated with unexplained infertility.* Hum Reprod, 2000. 15(5): p. 1046-51.

92. Bannatyne, P., P. Russell, and R.P. Shearman, *Autoimmune oophoritis: a clinicopathologic assessment of 12 cases.* Int J Gynecol Pathol, 1990. 9(3): p. 191-207.

93. Lahita, R.G., *Predisposing factors to autoimmune disease.* Int J Fertil Womens Med, 1997. 42(2): p. 115-9.

94. Olsen, N.J. and W.J. Kovacs, *Gonadal steroids and immunity.* Endocr Rev, 1996. 17(4): p. 369-84.

95. Goswami, R., *et al.*, *Pituitary autoimmunity in patients with Sheehan's syndrome.* J Clin Endocrinol Metab, 2002. 87(9): p. 4137-41.

96. Schrager, S. and L. Sabo, *Sheehan syndrome: a rare complication of postpartum hemorrhage.* J Am Board Fam Pract, 2001. 14(5): p. 389-91.

97. De Bellis, A.A., *et al.*, *Time course of 21-hydroxylase antibodies and long-term remission of subclinical autoimmune adrenalitis after corticosteroid therapy: case report.* J Clin Endocrinol Metab, 2001. 86(2): p. 675-8.

98. Orrego, J.J. and A.L. Barkan, *Pituitary disorders. Drug treatment options.* Drugs, 2000. 59(1): p. 93-106.

99. *And then there were none,* 2003, California Medical Association.

100. Burnum, J.F., *La maladie du petit papier. Is writing a list of symptoms a sign of an emotional disorder?* N Engl J Med, 1985. 313(11): p. 690-1.

101. Kelestimur, S., *The frequency of late-onset 21-hydroxylase and 11 beta-hydroxylase deficiency in women with polycystic ovarian syndrome.* Eur J Endocrinol, 1997. 137(6):670-4.

102. Jacobs, A, *et al. Late-onset congenital adrenal hyperplasia: a treatable cause of anxiety.* Biol Psychiatry. 1999. 46(6):856-9.

INDEX

A
adrenals
21-hydroxylase antibodies, 53
Addison's disease, 49
treatment, 54
hormones, 46
secondary insufficiency, 51
aldosterone, 46
B
bleeding, breakthrough, 122
C
chemicals
ovarian function effect, 92
converting lab data, 160
cortisol
adrenal, 46
salivary testing method, 59
treatment with, 54
Cushings' syndrome, 56
E
endometriosis, 86
autoimmune, 87
diagnosis, 89
symptoms, 88
treatment, 90
estradiol
PCOS treatment, 84
PMS therapy, 72
estrogen
formats, 111
levels during ovulation, 66
Euthyroid, sick thyroid syndrome, 23

F
FEMALE formula, 137
ferritin,
effect on thyroid medication, 35
menopause, 103
symptoms, 34
fibroids, 122
G
Graves' disease, 20
H
hair loss, 82
Hashimoto's disease, 17
treatment, 24
health scrapbook, 135
Hormones
abnormal cycle, 6
normal cycle, 1
see individual hormones
hormone therapy
route of administration, 111
Hyperthyroidism, treatment, 39
Hypothyroidism,
non-medication therapies, 37
I
insulin resistance
in PCOS, 78
L
late onset congenital adrenal hyperplasia, 79
list making, 133
M
medical records, collection 147
consent form, 149

medication
   dissolve under tongue, 118
menopause
   breakthrough bleeding, 122
   myths, 106
   premature, 127
   premenopause, 97
      symptoms, 99
      therapy, 101
      midcycle values, 104
   post, hormone therapies,
      111
   testing, 100
menstrual cycle
   charting symptoms, 8
   hormone levels, 66
   salivary levels, 68
   summary, 64

O
orthostatic hypotension, 50
ovarian cancer, 93
ovarian cysts, 85
Ovulation
   hormone levels, 2, 3
   sialic acid test, 5

P
PMS, 70
   hormone testing, 69
Polycystic ovarian syndrome, 74
   features, 76
   ring of cysts, 77
   treatment, 81

Polyglandular Autoimmune
   Disorder, 52
prednisone, 55
premature menopause, 127
   diagnostic lab studies, 129
progesterone, 3, 67
   salivary false reading, 68

R
rules of hormone interplay ,1
rules of negotiation, 131

T
T3, potency, 15
thumpies, 28
Thyroid
   adding T3 to medication, 29
   antibodies,
      selenium effect, 30
   function, 15
   hyperthyroid symptoms, 21
   hypothyroid symptoms, 13
   lab patterns, 17
   medications, 26
   nodules, 40
   test ranges, 12
tryptophan
   sources, 73

V
vaginal dryness, therapy, 125

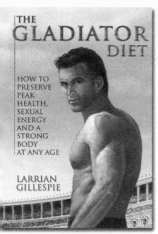

THE
GLADIATOR
DIET

HOW TO
PRESERVE
PEAK
HEALTH,
SEXUAL
ENERGY
AND A
STRONG
BODY
AT ANY AGE

LARRIAN
GILLESPIE

$17.95

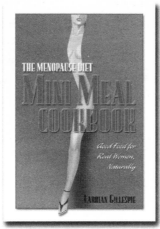

THE MENOPAUSE DIET
MINI MEAL
COOKBOOK

Good Food for
Real Women,
Naturally

LARRIAN GILLESPIE

$14.95

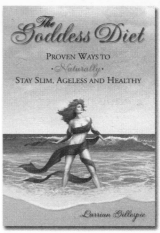

The
Goddess Diet

PROVEN WAYS TO
·Naturally·
STAY SLIM, AGELESS AND HEALTHY

Larrian Gillespie

$17.95

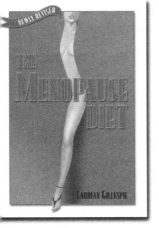

NEWLY REVISED

THE MENOPAUSE DIET

LARRIAN GILLESPIE

$19.95

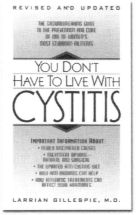

REVISED AND UPDATED

THE GROUNDBREAKING GUIDE
TO THE PREVENTION AND CURE
OF ONE OF WOMEN'S
MOST STUBBORN AILMENTS

YOU DON'T
HAVE TO LIVE WITH
CYSTITIS

IMPORTANT INFORMATION ABOUT:
• NEWLY DISCOVERED CAUSES
• TREATMENT OPTIONS—
  NATURAL AND SURGICAL
• THE UPDATED ANTI-CYSTITIS DIET
• HOW ANTI-OXIDANTS CAN HELP
• HOW ANTIBIOTIC TREATMENTS CAN
  AFFECT YOUR HORMONES

LARRIAN GILLESPIE, M.D.

$12.00

**"TOP 10
BESTSELLER"**

on women's health by
The New York Review of Books'
Reader's Catalog, 1999

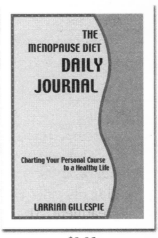

THE
MENOPAUSE DIET
DAILY
JOURNAL

Charting Your Personal Course
to a Healthy Life

LARRIAN GILLESPIE

$9.95

© 2003 Larrian Gillespie

Available in bookstores everywhere, or call 1-800-554-3335
for VISA or MasterCard orders. Prices do not include shipping.
Order online at www.menopausediet.com

Larrian Gillespie

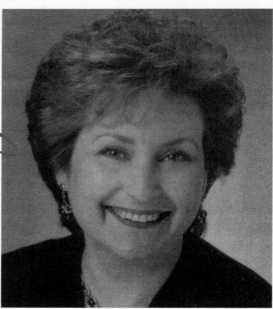

© 2003 Larrian Gillespie

LARRIAN GILLESPIE graduated from the
UCLA School of Medicine and retired as a
Clinical Assistant Professor of Urology and
Urogynecology in 1995. She is the inventor
on three drug patents.

Known for her ability to relay complicated
medical information in a patient friendly
manner, she has appeared on Good Morning
America, CNN and served on the advisory
board of SHAPE Magazine, Prevention Books
and Readers Digest Books. She has
published over fifty scientific articles and
three chapters in medical textbooks.

She is the author of "The Menopause Diet,"
"The Goddess Diet," The Menopause Diet
Mini Meal Cookbook," "The Menopause Diet
Daily Journal," "The Gladiator Diet," "You
Don't Have to Live With Cystitis," and
"You're Not Crazy It's Your Hormones."